Back Story

Back Story

BREAKING THE CYCLE OF CHRONIC PAIN

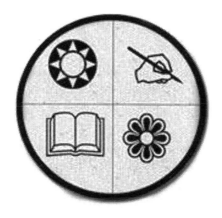

Zone Four Media
2015

Sherri A. Obermark

Printed in the United States of America
First Printing, January 2015

ISBN-13: 9780692304396 (Zone Four Media)
ISBN-10: 0692304398
Library of Congress Control Number: 2014953804
Zone Four Media, Cincinnati, Ohio

Zone Four Media
www.breakthecycleofchronicpain.com

Dedication

This book is dedicated to my father, Charles A. Briening, who was a smart, creative, funny, thoughtful, forward-looking, and kind man. He was an inspiration to everyone who knew him and a guiding light for me.

Table of Contents

Acknowledgments

WISH TO thank my parents, Fran and Charles, who taught me the value of hard work and persistence. Their inspiration has sustained me through difficult times, and allowed me to understand that almost any problem can be solved with imagination, patience, and logic.

To my sister, Mary, I am grateful for the example of her kindness, love, and grace. She will always be an inspiration to me.

My husband, Peter, provided steady guidance and helpful suggestions during the writing of this book. I could not have found a more supportive and loving partner with whom to walk through life.

Finally, my thanks to dear Nathan, you inspire so many people every day, and you are my hero!

What BACK STORY?
My BACK STORY.
Maybe your BACK STORY?

Introduction

THIS BOOK IS a description of my personal journey—from decades of musculoskeletal pain and discomfort to complete freedom from chronic pain. That may seem like a sweeping, even hyperbolic claim, but this experience has changed my entire understanding of health and fitness and has utterly transformed my outlook on life. It is this joy, exuberance, and relief that I hope to bring to everyone suffering from chronic musculoskeletal pain. If someone reads this book, learns from my experience, and achieves a measure of relief from his or her own chronic pain, then I will consider this modest project a success. I am fully aware that each person—each case—is different and that what has worked for me may not work for everyone in the same manner, but it is my hope that it will bring relief to many of you.

The proposition that physical and mental health are intertwined and that physical ailments can be exacerbated or even caused by emotional stress is now widely accepted as a general principal in both the mainstream and alternative medical communities.

This connection between physical and emotional health is a concept with deep roots in the history of medicine. Both Eastern and Western traditions in the ancient and early modern world—from Ayurveda traditions and Chinese medicine to classical Greek philosophers, such as Plato and Aristotle, and European intellectuals as diverse as Descartes and Kant—have speculated on the ways in which the health of mind and body are mutually dependent on one another.

Most of us already know that our minds and bodies are connected physiologically, but how and to what degree? In the hustle-bustle of our busy lives, it can be difficult for many of us to see how this connection may affect us from day to day.

After making some simple changes to my life, I now understand how profoundly the mind-body connection impacts us. For me, personally, the catalyst for writing this book was half a lifetime of chronic pain that was often near debilitating and robbed me of joy, energy, and a positive spirit.

For most of my adult life I was perfectly healthy, and capable of doing everything I wanted. Shortly after my 30th birthday, however, things changed suddenly and drastically as my body became afflicted with chronic musculoskeletal pain. At times, it was so severe that I found I was unable to sit or stand. It was frightening and baffling. What was happening to me? Initially the pain seemed mostly focused in my lower back, but later I would have bouts of chronic pain in my lower joints, including my hips, knees, and ankles. During these prolonged episodes of chronic pain, I wondered if I would be physically up for any type of excursion I wanted to plan. My husband and I love to hike. Whether we're at a local park; walking in cities like San Francisco, New Orleans, or London; or running along a beach in the Caribbean, we enjoy walking outdoors. When we were on our adventurous honeymoon in Alaska, I struggled with a swollen, aching ankle as we hiked through Denali National Park. Each evening, we would search for some ice to create a cold compress, trying to bring down the swelling in my foot and ankle in time for the next day's hike. I was suffering from one of my many pop-up strain-ache pains, which I endured for so many years. This was my normal daily routine, trying to make the pain go away long enough to do what I wanted or needed to do. Maybe it is part of your routine, too?

If I were to describe my pain, I would say it was like a multiheaded hydra, with various types of agonizing discomforts. Once the pain began, it was almost always accompanied by a dull ache in my lower back, or sometimes it would be in a different part of my body. There was an array of pains: a burning sensation, a stabbing pain, a spiky pain, a lightning bolt of pain, a tearing pain, a pulling pain, a twisting pain, an uncomfortable heat, and the feeling of smoldering hot coals sitting just under the skin of my lower back.

As I reflect on what I endured, I think I should've been able to understand that my problem was not some specific injury, because if it were just one injury, logically I would always have a similar pain in a similar place. Truthfully, it wasn't always in the same place—it changed, it became something else, and it was always transient. The pain varied in its intensity; sometimes it was bad enough to stop me from going to work or even getting out of bed. Other times it was just a small, annoying, and constant reminder that all was not well in my bones and joints. I would later discover that it had nothing to do with the bones or joints themselves, but at the time, that is what I believed.

I would become despondent during severe episodes. Sometimes the pain was so intense that I was unable to even stand up without assistance. At those times, I was so distracted that I could barely open a book or even summon a sufficient attention span to listen to the radio or watch a television show. At night I couldn't sleep because there was no position that was comfortable, and my mind would race with recurring anxieties about what would happen to me: Would I be able to work again? Would I lose my house? Where would this end?

In the middle of a particularly bad, spasming LBP (low-back pain) event, I spent the better part of an hour gingerly sliding myself out of bed, wincing and shouting in agony as I eased myself onto the floor and crawled across the hall to the desk where I keep important papers. I struggled to get to the files I was seeking and then reviewed my short-term and long-term disability insurance policies, which was something I had never felt the need to do in the past. Suddenly, understanding how to submit a disability claim, and what I could expect in terms of benefits, was very important. I was trying to imagine what kind of life I would have if I could never work again. There may never have been another time in my life when I felt as lost and alone as I did at that moment.

During those dark times I did not know whom to turn to for help. I have a wonderful, supportive family, and they knew that I had back pain, but they never knew how bad it was, and I did not want to dump all my fears and troubles on them. I was seeking the best medical care I could find, and I had some help from some very caring health-care providers over the years, but none of them had the answers for me.

These occasions of excruciating pain were truly terrifying for me and included a dangerous instability in my entire trunk, pelvis, and legs. I often felt as though I would crumble, that my body would be permanently broken, that I would be changed forever, and that I would never stand or walk again. During these times, I suddenly felt fragile, when I had never been that way before. This progression was completely puzzling to me, because I had always been strong and capable of doing whatever physical tasks I wanted to achieve. Looking back on that time, I now realize I was never seriously harmed, although everything I felt made me believe otherwise.

Today, it seems strange to me that I truly believed I was permanently disabled and had been told by many doctors that, essentially, I had a soft-tissue injury that would not *ever* heal, an injury that I would always have. Happily, none of those things were true; there was nothing seriously wrong with me, even when I felt barely capable of standing. I was as capable as I had ever been, except for these strange pains that seemed to come from nowhere—and for which, I was told, there was no cure. I later found that all of my pain was the result of a condition that continually caused injury to my body. Until I removed that condition, I was always going to be in pain.

If you have chronic pain, you know that there is almost nothing you won't try to make yourself feel better, and I tried pretty much everything. I looked at every part of my life and attempted to find a way to make myself comfortable, and in the process, I discovered just how creative I could be.

Work is a big part of my life, so of course I tried every imaginable ergonomic set-up for my desk and my computer chair. I tried a ball chair, a footstool that pivoted, and pillows. I tried a hard, wooden chair, and every type of ergonomic chair I could find. I set my chair back up straight and then so it would allow me to flex backward. I used a platform to raise and lower the keyboard, mouse, and monitor. I even tried a standing desk. If it was out there in the marketplace, I tried it to make my pain tolerable during the workday. None of it helped.

In my attempts to relax at home, I tried sitting on the couch or a hardback chair with a pillow behind my back, sitting on a pillow on a chair, and sitting on a pillow on the floor. None of these things made me more comfortable.

The car was another environment I had to endure with my chronic back pain. I tried putting a pillow on the seat, sitting with a small pillow behind my back—or maybe a bigger pillow—and then I'd try no pillow at all. I would move the seat all the way back and then all the way forward. I'd adjust the back of the seat so it was straight up and down and then try reclining it. If I was having a complete low-back spasm, getting in or out of the car could be a fifteen-minute ordeal. I'd carefully slide into the front seat and try to swing both my legs together, which made the pain worse.

Even walking and standing is painful when you have chronic pain, so footwear is important. I tried hard-soled shoes, new running shoes with lots of cushioning, and barefoot-type running shoes, and of course I had to say good-bye to high heels.

Finding a comfortable way to sleep was another battle. I tried sleeping with one pillow below my head, two pillows below my head, a flat pillow, or sometimes a puffy pillow. I put a pillow between my knees and another one between my ankles. I might have a long body pillow to lean against, and then maybe I'd feel like I needed to have another pillow behind my back. Then I'd feel that none of that was working, and I'd start removing the pillows. After that I'd start to think about buying myself a new mattress.

Trying to operate in the world when you are suffering from chronic pain comes down to an endless series of adjustments and accommodations, but few bring us comfort, and none bring us a cure. When I think about all of the time energy, effort, and money that I've spent to lessen my chronic pain, it makes me very sad. If only I had known about TMR (Total Muscular Release), I could've saved myself an enormous amount of pain and trouble. I hope that some of you reading this will find relief from what I will share in this book.

Chronic neck, back, shoulder, or any other debilitating pain leaves the victim in severe agony. It is a misery that I experienced. It is intense, and it is *real*. Chronic pain can morph from an ache to a burning sensation or uncomfortable spasms; or from soreness into a nearly convulsive state of pain. At times I was completely obsessed with finding a relief from the discomfort, which was my torturous companion for years.

In the following pages, I will describe how my chronic low-back pain appeared seemingly out of the blue; how this condition negatively impacted my life; how I spent long years attempting to fix the problem; what I ultimately learned about my condition; and how I was able to create a cure that brought me peace and a blissful end to twenty years of chronic back pain.

What did this *cure* require of me? I had to come to understand that my mind was causing the physical pain in my body on a subconscious level and, most importantly, that there was something I could do about it. I had to come up with a plan of action and follow through with it. I had to put time and energy into this healing method even though, at first, I wasn't really sure if it would work for me. Once I was committed to these concepts and efforts, there was nothing else to do but move ahead. I had tried everything else, so what did I have to lose?

What did I get for my efforts? In short order, everything changed for me in a wonderful and exciting way. I reached the end of years of crippling chronic pain; I discovered a true understanding of how the mind controls the body—really controls it; and I found a method for managing the situation in the future. Once I gained the knowledge of how to relax my body and deal with my emotions, I was completely free and able to control my present and future life. There was an absolute *eureka* moment when I realized that nearly everything I had been told about my chronic pain was wrong—just flat-out wrong.

As I sit here at my desk, writing this book for hours at a time, I think, *How is it possible that I am capable of doing this when, just a year ago, I would have had to jump up out of my seat after twenty minutes from the agonizing pain in my back and down through my legs?* My work life of testing computer systems and writing had long been a constant struggle between duty and pain. I understood that I had obligations to my coworkers and employer to get my work done, but I often found myself distracted by the discomfort.

Though many normal daily tasks caused me trepidation, there was no activity that I dreaded as much as sitting in an economy seat on a commercial flight for hours and hours. We traveled to Kauai, Hawaii, which is truly one of the loveliest places on earth, but the thirteen-hour multileg flight to get there was a study in pain and frustration. As the time crawled by, I wished that I could get up and walk off the plane, which is a difficult thing to do at thirty thousand feet in the air. I struggled with a constant pulling sensation from my back down into my pelvis, and endless tightening in my calves and ankles.

Happily, these days I no longer fear a short flight, long flight, or any trip for that matter, because I know I can control my tension and stop my pain before it starts. A recent trip to the UK was completely pain-free, and it allowed me to sleep and rest, which is a thing I could never do with chronic pain.

Do I sometimes feel a bit of tightness or pain creeping into my back or my knee? Yes, it happens, but now I know that I can take control, relax my muscles, and make the pain fade and disappear. It is empowering to recognize that I have the power to control my mind and body, and this knowledge gives me a feeling of freedom I have found nowhere else.

I'm sure you're thinking that this all sounds too easy to be true. How can this simple method resolve your chronic pain? The concepts are not complex, but you will need to tailor them to your individual situation. You are the only one who can do this work, so stick with it until it is second nature, and with determination you too can manage your tension and be pain-free once again.

Perhaps you are thinking, *Why should I listen to this person? She isn't a doctor, chiropractor, or even a physical therapist.* It's true that I have no medical training, and I am not suggesting any medical intervention. I have referenced many medical-research and peer-reviewed studies concerning back-pain treatment, as well as the cause of chronic low-back pain, which support my assertions. If you have had chronic pain for a long time and have attempted to find a medical solution, you probably know that most doctors don't have an easy cure. So why not give this a try?

You will certainly want to read further if your situation is like mine: you've seen the doctor/sports-medicine practitioner/chiropractor, had the x-ray/MRI, gone to therapy, had acupuncture, taken up yoga and exercise classes, bought a special pillow-chair-mattress, etc., but you are still suffering from chronic back-neck-shoulder or other pain. What has worked so well for me—what I am proposing here—is simple; it's free, you can learn it here in these pages, and it's an intrinsic ability you have within you right now. You only need to understand and apply it.

Living for decades with chronic pain has left me with a lot of regret. It's not just that I didn't know what I needed to know to make myself better, or that I missed out on many things I could have enjoyed. There's also the feeling that I may have missed out on many more things I didn't even know about, because so often I didn't feel well enough to get up and see friends, meet people, and try new things. Experiences I didn't have because I was too busy dealing with my pain.

Why did I suffer with chronic low-back pain all those years? Why did I have to struggle like that? Why was no one able to help me? I ask myself these questions often, and the only response I have is that in the end, *I alone* had the answer. All of that lost time is my greatest regret.

Maybe I can save some of you from that regret. I hope you will learn about this method, find relief, and enjoy your lives. If some of you who are sufferers of chronic pain can learn to free yourselves from your pain through my story, which would be a great gift to me. It would help to make me feel that a lot of my suffering was somehow worthwhile.

■ ■ ■

The Reason: Chronic Pain

WHY DID I feel the need to write this book? I wanted to share my very surprising and incredible experience with others who suffer from chronic pain. I know what it feels like to be hopeless when it comes to chronic pain. I wish I had known about the cause of muscle tension ten, fifteen, or twenty years ago. In these pages, I hope to make these concepts simple to understand so others can easily apply these methods to their lives to resolve their pain. After taking this journey, it is clear to me that I was a sufferer of *tension myositis syndrome* (TMS). Tension was created in my back muscles, the contracted muscles were starved of oxygen, and that resulted in pain, which became chronic over time. After gaining the basic premise of the theory put forth by Dr. John Sarno, a physician who's book "Healing Back Pain: The Mind-Body Connection" provided important insights for me, I was able to develop a method to resolve my crippling pain. In little more than a few weeks, practicing a series of disciplines allowed me to break the cycle of tension, and I was pain-free. It is my genuine and sincere hope that this knowledge can yield the same results for readers.

Pain in the back, neck, or shoulders can have many causes, such as infection, trauma, cancer, severe osteoporosis, or other illness that may need medical intervention, and a full workup by a trained health-care professional is required for anyone suffering from pain. Those experiencing back, neck, shoulder, or any other intense pain should be seen by a medical professional to rule out any serious medical issue.

If there is no serious, organic medical issue at hand, that is when the search for relief begins. Sometimes the patient is given some vague diagnosis: "You may have a *pinched nerve*," "You may have a *compressed disc*," "You may have intervertebral *disc degeneration*," etc. These kinds of suggestions seem like a lot of conjecture with no real traceable cause and effect for the discomfort. Many people have these very same conditions by a certain age, but experience no pain. After struggling with and enduring excruciating pain for so long, I found very little solace in these nebulous responses. They were giving me their best answers I'm sure, but they never satisfied me.

When we look at the state of diagnosis and treatment for back pain, we see that, after several decades of study, there is very little in terms of concrete diagnoses for the ailing back-pain patient. This will be discussed further in the chapter Current Scientific Research on Chronic Back-Pain.

Getting a clear diagnosis is difficult, if not impossible, but finding a concise treatment plan for back-neck-shoulder pain can be even more confusing to patients. Patients suffering from back pain are prescribed a myriad of treatment options, such as hot compresses, cold compresses, rest, exercise, pain medication, chiropractic care, intradiscal electrothermal therapy (IDET), bioelectric therapy, nerve blocks, spinal stimulation, back surgery, acupuncture, transcutaneous electrical nerve stimulation (TENS), steroid injections, physical therapy, and on and on. Suffers may also find themselves confused by the information they receive from well-meaning friends, family, neighbors, and co-workers offering endless cures, suggestions, and home remedies.

For many, the hunt continues for a resolution to their pain. A search of YouTube today for back-pain relief exercises yielded 192,000 results.

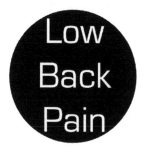

A search of YouTube today for neck-pain relief exercises displayed 104,000 results.

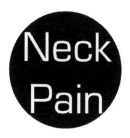

A search of YouTube today for sciatica pain-relief exercises displayed 103,000 results.

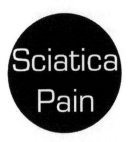

Clearly, an enormous amount of energy must go into developing, writing, producing, and uploading hundreds of thousands of videos to YouTube and other websites. It is obvious from the results shown in three single categories on just one website that there is a great demand for relief from back, neck, and sciatica pain. The search for a cure is obviously incessant, as there are so many people desperate for relief.

Of course, doctors are doing their best to treat their patients who come to them in a frenzied state of pain. Dr. John Sarno, who first identified TMS, describes his early experiences of treating patients with back, neck, and shoulder pain as being depressing and frustrating, because regardless of the treatment that was applied, he could never be certain what would work for whom and for how long. Doubtless there are numerous medical practitioners who cannot heal many of their chronic-pain patients and feel this same dissatisfaction.

According to the National Center for Complementary and Alternative Medicine (NCCAM), a part of the US Department of

Health and Human Services National Institutes of Health, the total annual cost for people with low-back pain in the United States is more than 100 billion dollars, which includes lost wages and reduced employee productivity. Back pain is one of the most common health complaints and affects eight out of ten people during their lives, with the lower back often the most affected area. The pain may go away on its own; however, for some people, the pain becomes chronic and may last for months, years, or even decades. Lower-back pain may be very debilitating, and it is a condition that is challenging to diagnose, treat, and study.

My own search for relief from chronic back pain involved dozens of healthcare professionals, hundreds of lost hours of work and family life, and thousands of dollars in treatments and medications over decades, without even the smallest hint of how I could resolve my pain. I would often ask myself as the years went by, *How is it possible that all this time and money and these resources, tests, and treatments could lead to little or no tangible result?*

My personal experience led me to understand that there was no medical treatment, or external physical intervention, that could have cured my back or knee pain. Some interventions did make me feel better for a period of time, but eventually they all failed to bring me lasting relief. The therapeutics I tried, regardless of the type of modality, were doing only one thing for me, and that was bringing blood flow and oxygen to my long-suffering, contracted muscles. As soon as the therapy stopped, the muscles contracted once again and were again starved for oxygen, and needless to say the pain returned. The pain I was feeling was physical in nature but was driven by an internal source, which would continue to make me suffer until I dealt with the issues. Once my *emotional* energy was under control, I was able to manage my own *physical* environment.

During the most harrowing battles with chronic low-back pain, I lost productive time in my life, which I regret every minute of, but I didn't have the knowledge to change it. If anyone reading this can save themselves from losing days, weeks, months, or years of their lives to chronic pain by using the methods described in the following chapters, I will be humbled and pleased beyond measure.

Again, I am not a medical doctor, and I cannot diagnose anyone else's pain; but I will describe how making some simple changes could potentially help others free themselves from pain.

■ ■ ■

Pain and the Search for Healing

LMOST EVERYONE SUFFERS from low-back pain at some point in his or her life. According to the US National Institutes of Health (NIH), Americans spend an estimated 50 billion to 100 billion dollars on diagnosing and treating lower-back pain each year. It is the leading cause of missed workdays and job-related disability, and it is the second most common neurological disorder in the United States, after headaches. Low-back pain occurrences are often gone within a few days, but for some of us, the pain becomes chronic, with *chronic pain* being described as lasting three months or more. The symptoms of low-back pain may be muscle aches, spasms, and shooting or stabbing pains, which greatly limit flexibility and range of motion. Sometimes the pain will radiate to other parts of the body, the pain may be referential, or it may move through the body.

During my long battle with chronic low-back and other musculoskeletal pain, I suffered from all of these symptoms: muscle aches, spasms, and shooting or stabbing pains, radiating pain, and referential pain before I learned a way out. The good news is there may be a pain-free pathway forward for you in the future, even if you have pain in many parts of your body. I found this path, and I hope you will too.

Below you will find a short biological primer about the human back. The back contains five different regions:

- the seven cervical or neck vertebrae (C1–C7)
- the twelve thoracic or upper-back vertebrae (T1–T12)
- the five lumbar vertebrae (L1–L5)
- the lower-back and pelvic-area sacrum
- the coccyx (which is fused with the sacrum at the base of the spine)

The Cervical

The seven vertebrae in the neck make up the cervical section of the spine. The cervical vertebrae are the thinnest and most delicate vertebrae found in the spine, which allows the neck to have the necessary flexibility. The C1 vertebra supports the skull, which pivots on the atlas when moving up and down. The C2 vertebra is known as the *axis* and allows the skull left and right rotation.

The Thoracic

The chest area consists of twelve vertebrae, which comprise the spine's thoracic area. These vertebrae are stronger and larger than cervical vertebrae but also are much less flexible. The thoracic vertebrae form a joint with each pair of ribs, creating a strong rib cage to protect the organs located within the chest cavity.

The Lumbar

The lumbar area consists of five vertebrae comprising the lower-back region of the spine. These vertebrae are stronger and even larger than the thoracic vertebrae but have more flexibility because they are not connected to ribs like the thoracic vertebrae. The lumbar vertebrae carry most of the weight of the upper body.

The Sacral

The sacral region involves just the sacrum, which is a single bone in adults and is formed by the fusion of five smaller vertebrae after adolescence. The triangular-shaped sacrum is flat and found in the lower back between the hipbones.

The Coccygeal

The coccygeal section has only the single coccyx bone in the adult spine and is formed after childhood by the fusion of four tiny vertebrae similar to the sacral. Most people know the coccyx as the tailbone. The coccyx supports our body weight when we sit and provides a place to attach the muscles of the pelvic and gluteal areas.

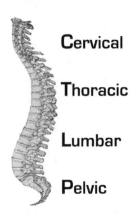

Cervical

Thoracic

Lumbar

Pelvic

Returning to my story, I had lower-back pain for about twenty years. It was awful, came out of nowhere, and scared the hell out of me. But it was miraculously gone ten days or so after I discovered and practiced the method described in the pages below.

I was generally healthy and pain-free into my early thirties. When my troubles began, I was working with computers at a financial data–services company in Bethesda, Maryland. One day I walked out of my office building and found myself looking at the sky. I'd stumbled and sprained my right ankle quite badly. It took about a month before I could drive again and get my life back to normal. Shortly after that sprain, I began to have a series of physical problems that I had never previously experienced before.

It's important to stop here and examine the course of events I experienced, as well as the narrative I created to understand why these things began to happen to me. I had heard stories from family and friends about injuries that they'd had as a kid or an adult, and how those damaging events from the past continued to cause them pain for years.

I'd had a bad sprain, that is true, but sprains usually heal completely, and they don't morph into leg, knee, hip, and back pain. I'd heard the theory about ligaments and tendons being stretched, or out of alignment. In order to explain these issues, I created a "Pain Story" for myself, about a sprain causing a misalignment in my body, which was the cause of all these other pain issues. I've since learned that none of this was true, but at the time it seemed reasonable. The mind wants to understand what is going on, and if it can't get the real story, sometimes it does some *creative* writing. I told my theory to many doctors over the years, and none of them ever corrected me or told me that my pain story was implausible.

Maybe you have created a Pain Story to help explain why you were suffering; perhaps you have even repeated it to others. But please take some time to consider that your Pain Story may not be exactly what you think it is.

Shortly after the sprain, I began to experience a sort of pulling pain down the front of my right calf, but it felt like it was near the bone. It seemed like a serious issue, and I imagined it was a problem with a vein in my right leg. After a doctor ruled out any vein issues, I attributed that discomfort to tight calf muscles.

I read up on tightened calf muscles and found the universal opinion was that sitting too much at a desk caused the condition. There are many resources on the Internet describing the aliment of shortened calf muscles and offering exercises to correct it. Some websites described the calf muscles as "notorious" for shortening, and I remember thinking it sounded strange that these muscles could become shortened, as no other muscles seem to have this problem.

I worked with computers and systems, which required me to sit in front of a computer for most of the day. Since I'd been doing this work for a long time, I couldn't understand why I'd never had this issue before. I would rub my calf, ankle, and foot at the end of the day to make them feel better, but it provided only temporary relief.

Today there is no need to spend hours every week working my calf muscles with stretching exercises, as I once did, because I don't have shortened calf muscles—and I never did have them. I had a condition that caused the calf muscles to tighten, and I'm happy to say I have conquered that now.

During recent decades, I've had many physical complaints, which I now attribute to TMS. I had hip, pelvic, and ankle pain; plantar fasciitis; other leg-based aches and pains; and an intractable case of sciatica. I had back pain year after year, and I also experienced severe knee pain for approximately three years. All of these pains came and went at different times, sometimes for weeks, months, or years, for no understandable reason. There *was*, of course, an understandable reason for all of these pains; I simply did not have that knowledge.

At one point, I started a jogging program, which I enjoyed. Soon after that, however, I began to experience hip pain during or after a run. Sometimes it was the right hip, sometimes the left hip, and sometimes both hips. Sometimes it was just an annoyance, but other times it was so bad I had to stop jogging and walk the rest of the way. I tried some over-the-counter balms and rubs but never had any lasting relief from them. When the hip pain began, I would often also experience pelvic pain, which was achy and sort of moved around. The hip pain and the corresponding pelvic pain were intermittent, and I didn't understand why.

Chronic pain sometimes made me too timid to try new things because I believed that my body was in a vulnerable state, and if I pushed myself I would undoubtedly be hurt in some way. I've since discovered that I wasn't in any sort of delicate, breakable state—I was under physical stress from an internal source.

If you've ever had sciatica, you know that it can be maddening, painful, debilitating, confounding, and almost impossible to resolve. In 2008, when I had my first brush with sciatica, I was amazed that something as prevalent as sciatica could be so poorly understood. I found that no one seemed to know how it started, how to treat it, what made it better or worse, how it could be resolved, why certain people were afflicted with it, or how it was resolved. My bout with sciatica, which was approximately six months in duration, came completely out of the blue and lasted for what felt like forever, although I later discovered it was not a terribly long time in terms of what others have suffered. I was shocked to learn that some people's sciatica essentially never goes away.

It started when I woke up one day with severe back pain, and at first I thought it was just another series of lower-right-back spasms, which was something I had endured many times before. I wondered if this was just going to be the usual discomfort, or if would it bloom into a spasming episode that would render me incapable of living my life.

Eventually the pain started to change, and it migrated down into my pelvis on the right and sort of ricocheted around back and forth between my hips, which created an awful feeling of instability in my trunk. Over time the pain settled into my left leg at the hip. This was new—and not an encouraging development. This pain is hard to describe, except to say that it felt like the tendons in my thigh were being roughly pulled up and through my leg. Sometimes it was dull ache radiating up or down my body; sometimes it was a stabbing pain; and sometimes it felt like a lightning bolt.

The pain almost never stopped and seemed to be with me every moment of the day and night. I would dream about being in pain and wake up to find, indeed, I was in agony. My work was beginning to suffer because I had trouble staying still in my chair while trying to find some tolerable position. For many months, there was no position while sitting, standing, walking, or lying down in which I felt at peace.

There was no end to my efforts to stop the pain of sciatica. I went to my chiropractor, who had helped me with back pain in the past, week-in and week-out for months. I tried acupuncture for the first time. I did exercises three or four times per day. I stretched every way I could think to do so. I did endless abdominal work—crunches, leg lifts, and yoga—and even bought an inversion table. I walked and walked around the neighborhood every day and hoped that I could somehow walk out the pain. Even though every step hurt me, I knew that *not* moving would be worse than being active.

When I was sleepless and awake at two or three o'clock in the morning, I had a lot of time to fill, so I searched for answers on the Internet. I spent countless hours trying different search terms to find the answers to what causes sciatica and, most importantly, what I could do to resolve it. A search of Google for "sciatica" at the time yielded about 2,880,000 results. Where to start? There are so many theories, ideas, and thoughts on the subject and thousands of anecdotal stories about people who did this or tried that and somehow got relief, but there is no consensus, and nothing concrete.

I was always fascinated with the personal stories and would spend hours reading medical message boards to see what people had to say. When I was searching at that time, I really wanted to find that woman or man who had a story just like mine, someone with a similar lifestyle, job, background, or symptoms. Maybe that person would have the exact set of exercises, stretches, treatments, or whatever I needed to make myself better. I might have considered voodoo or a magic potion at that point if I thought it would help me.

My research led me to the conclusion that the medical community really had no solid answers as to the cause of sciatica or what would constitute effective treatment for it. How, after so many years, could so many learned people be so clueless about a condition so prevalent in our society? I read many vague theories about pinched nerves; pulled muscles; deteriorated discs; and body-alignment, posture, and breathing issues.

I read about problems with the piriformis muscle, which, according to Wikipedia, is the pear-shaped muscle in the gluteal region of the lower limb and is one of the six muscles in the lateral rotator. I had never heard of it before. The piriformis muscle, which is buried deep in the musculature of the pelvis, is something I soon began to read a lot about. Some friends told me they thought the piriformis was a potential cause of their sciatica pain, but I never heard about any treatment for the piriformis that cured sciatica. Why would that tiny little muscle, quiet for all those years, suddenly go on the fritz with no logical cause? It made no sense to me.

The NIH is a fine institution, but I've found it quite telling that this organization reflects a lot of the confusion about disorders, such as sciatica, in the medical community. On the very same web page, it describes sciatica as a symptom of problems with the sciatic nerve, and it also says that sciatica is caused by ruptured intervertebral discs, spinal stenosis, and pelvic fractures. It goes on to say that, in many cases, there is no cause to be found, and sometimes sciatica resolves itself.[1]

---

1 . Sciatica, http://www.nlm.nih.gov/medlineplus/sciatica.html.

Some pages I reviewed said that exercises, medicines, and surgery might be needed as treatment.[2]

As a person looking for answers to sciatica and reading that it may be caused by a nerve problem, ruptured intervertebral disc, spinal stenosis, pelvic fractures, or have no cause, and may be treated with exercises, medicines, surgery, or no intervention at all, I found neither surety nor comfort. Feeling as bad and hopeless as I did at the time, more uncertainty was the last thing I needed. Sitting in the dark, in what felt like my darkest hour, and reading stories about people who *never* get better and were cursed with the pain of sciatica for the rest of their lives, I feared the worst for my life and future.

Not knowing what else to do, I decided it was best for me to keep moving, as sitting, lying, or standing were all uncomfortable. So I set out on a program of walking every day—no excuses—just to be able to keep the blood circulating and the air moving in and out of my lungs. Sometimes I would walk a couple of miles at a time; sometimes I would be in too much pain, have no energy, and could only do a mile or less. At times I would feel pretty good and could easily move through my day, but other days were just brutal. I'd wake up in pain and not have a minute of the day without that searing hurt running across my body and down my leg.

After about four months, the pain slowly began to migrate down into my thigh, through the middle of my femur, and into my knee. I wasn't quite sure what to think of that, but it made sitting and lying down a little more comfortable, so I considered it a positive improvement. In the weeks that followed, it traveled down into my calf—aching with every step—and continued down into my ankle,

---

2 . NIH Low-Back Pain Fact Sheet, http://www.ninds.nih.gov/disorders/backpain/detail_backpain.htm.

and eventually into my foot. One day I woke up and felt, for the first time in a long time, no sciatica pain. But I was sure it would be back.

Looking over the many episodes of crippling pain I've experienced over the years, I now understand that those events clearly took place at times of high stress in my life. If I looked at the stressful events and periods in my life, I could almost chart it directly to physical pain events. We always have some kind of stress in our lives, but there are times when those emotions become more than we can handle, and we are not aware when we've reached our breaking point.

When we reach a point of overload, our minds have to do something with all of that overflowing energy and anxiety, and what it does is disperse it to other parts of our bodies. That displaced energy causes tension, which causes muscles to tighten, followed by a lack of oxygen to those muscles, and that is what brings us the dreaded pain. Much of that emotion is at a subconscious level, so we are not really aware of it. It is one of the reasons these sudden flare-ups of pain are so surprising. It is very important to be aware of what is going on in our thoughts, recent events that may have annoyed us, and situations which we are mentally grappling with.

As I reflect back, it is clear to me that my emotional states—not a sprain I experienced twenty years ago, regardless of my previous assertions—were most likely the cause of many of the physical issues I endured. I was in a difficult emotional place with a incompatible spouse, I had a very high-pressure job, and I had concerns about aging or ill parents and family members.

Even when a few years later, my marriage ended, and I had moved on to a new job, the pain did not dissipate. Instead, it morphed into new and sometimes different complaints because a pattern had been set. My autonomic nervous system knew that it had an outlet for unresolved feelings and emotions. My brain continued to deal with stress by causing tension in my body, which reduced the blood flow to those regions and continued to cause pain. This was a well-established pattern that truly haunted me for many years—a completely inscrutable chronic *loop*.

If you are reading this book, do not give up hope! I was in a terrible situation at the time, but I found my way out, and if you are in a similar state, you too can find your way to a place where you are no longer ruled by your pain.

My healing started during the winter of 2013–2014 in an out-of-the-blue sort of way. The season was a very rough one for southeastern Ohio, as it was for much of the country. It was ranked as the third snowiest season in recorded history, with 46.9 inches of snow, which included a killer snowstorm named Janus, and brutally cold temperatures in January and February. The birds and animals were hungry, and the trees and plants suffered, as did all of the two-legged inhabitants of the region. The snow started right after Thanksgiving and continued into April. I'm originally from New York, so I had seen a lot of cold temperatures, snow, and ice as I was growing up and throughout my adult life. That kind of weather didn't make much difference to me, generally, but that fierce winter seemed very different somehow.

During that time I felt as though I were in a frozen rut with constant back and knee pain and various and sundry other pains throughout my body from which I could not escape. Whatever method I tried, I could not get warm. Hot baths, layers and layers of clothing, endless cups of hot tea—nothing worked. I didn't want to go out to the track to run or even take a walk in the woods with my husband, which is something I enjoyed.

Traveling into the office felt like an enormous burden. I normally parked ten to twelve minutes from the building where I worked so I could get a quick walk in at the beginning and end of my day.

Suddenly I was parking a short block away and feeling even that was too much to ask.

The cold made me very sleepy, and it seemed to take my energy. I napped a lot, which is a thing I never did regularly before. I began to worry that I might have fibromyalgia or some similar illness, and that I had turned a very bad corner in my life. At the time, I had just entered my fifties and thought, *Is this it? Is this the way I will feel every day for the rest of my life? Will I always be in pain? Will it just get worse year after year, and is this what the future holds for me?*

Thankfully, I found a way to ensure my life would be free from chronic pain, and that pain was not going to be the final chapter in my story.

■ ■ ■

Introduction to TMR

T HE BEGINNING OF my cure came to me without any great fanfare: a story about back pain and tension on the radio one afternoon got my attention in an urgent sort of way, and I wanted to know more. The story described how tension could be the cause of chronic back, neck, and shoulder pain. That little news story got me thinking about my own tension and various pains and set me off to researching the connection between emotion, tension, and back-neck-shoulder pain. I knew tension was my problem, but I didn't know I could do anything about it. I discovered the work of Dr. John Sarno and his truly revolutionary thinking about the source of chronic pain. I quickly read through three of Dr. Sarno's books. His concept of tension myositis syndrome was understandable to me, and it seemed completely reasonable and solid in my mind. His explanation of how pain continued in a chronic state was the only interpretation of the issue I had ever heard that resonated with me.

If the largest bone in the body, the femur, is broken, it takes only approximately six weeks to heal. Why would a soft-tissue injury like a pulled muscle go on for years and years? I seemed to have an ongoing injury that went on for decades, but maybe it was just that those muscles were continuously under attack—under continuous tension. The reason for the tension is messaging from our subconscious mind telling our bodies to make those muscles tense. It might be difficult to hear that our own minds may be causing this pain week after week, month after month, year after year. We have seen the enemy, and it is us; but take heart—we can become friends, or at least reach an accord.

That all sounds pretty ominous at first, but there are really solid reasons for this phenomenon, and there is a cure. Muscle tension is a coping mechanism, which explains why it continues to cause us pain for long periods of time. When we have stress, and negative emotions that are not well managed, we may continue to have pain. My basic understanding of the function of TMS is as follows:

1. The subconscious mind must deal with a lot of difficult and negative emotional energy.
2. That energy can be released in the form of tension messages, which are transmitted to certain muscles in the body.
3. Those target muscles are contracted.
4. Blood flow is restricted.
5. The muscles are starved for oxygen.
6. Pain is perceived.

These emotions may be anger, disappointment, fear, stress, etc. Modern society often requires us to keep our negative emotions in check because expressing them out loud is not considered civil or appropriate behavior.

The subconscious mind must deal with these emotions somehow, so the autonomic nervous system (ANS) steps in to help relieve some of the emotional tension. One of the ANS's many tasks is to help us dissipate negative emotional energy, and in the process, there may be a disruption to the flow of blood, therefore limiting oxygen to the muscles. These muscles starved for oxygen begin to spasm and become nonfunctional, and this is the point where we have severe pain. When there is a large emotional load (stress, perhaps), suddenly we may experience an acute attack of pain described as "pulling" something in our back or "throwing out" our back. When this negative functioning of the autonomic nervous system continues over a long period of time, the pain will become chronic.

This syndrome theory seemed completely plausible to me, and I somehow knew that this was the basis of my problem. I had been to the chiropractor so often and heard the question so many times: "Do you know how tight your lower back muscles are?" Yes, yes, I knew I had tight muscles, but *why*? Why, indeed. In different therapeutic settings over decades, I had been told that I was sitting too much; I had bad posture; there was an issue with the way I was walking or a problem with the height of my desk, chair, computer monitor, or keyboard; my back, abs, and side muscles were weak; I needed to do some new exercise and stretch more; I needed to do more yoga; and on and on. All of those things seemed like a series of guesses or excuses and never really made sense to me, but this tension theory was the first logical explanation I had ever heard. Even though I was still in pain, I felt very excited at that point because I just knew there was an answer for me here.

You may be eager to find out what TMR is before I go into more detail below, so here is a list of concepts to review and, hopefully, embrace so that you can begin to eliminate tension and break the cycle of chronic pain in your body. These may seem like simple actions, but they may be the start of big changes for you. It will be important for you to accept all these concepts and work through the exercises in order for you to see the benefits. First believe that it is possible for your pain to be caused by tension, that the tension is caused by your mind, and that you can do something to break this pattern.

Practice Total Muscular Release

Follow this quick set of steps to achieve Total Muscular Release:

1. Lie down on your bed, couch, or yoga mat (whatever is the most comfortable for you), and begin to let your target muscles relax.
2. Make your target muscles drop completely to the surface that you are lying on.
3. Relax the surrounding muscles near your target muscles.
4. Understand your body will fight this because it is used to being in a tension state, so don't give up; keep releasing your target muscles.
5. This practice is not necessarily easy, but continue it until you can relax those muscles at will—do not quit.
6. Practice Total Muscular Release as often as you can, wherever you are. Make it a regular part of your daily routine.
7. Break the lock on those tense muscles, and allow them to relax—let go.
8. Practice Complete Release TMR for your whole body, from head to toe. Use self-talk while you work each muscle group.
9. Practice Active Total Muscular Release when you are moving, exercising, or other physical activity.

Self-talk

Talk to yourself silently or out loud—yell it out loud if you like—and tell your brain that there will be *no more* tension and *no more* pain in your target muscles. You may use any phrases that help you tell your mind and body what you expect. Use self-talk as you complete your whole-body TMR, while you release each muscle set.

Don't hold in your negative emotions

Don't keep negative emotions and feelings bottled up inside yourself. Express your feelings to others in an honest and nonthreatening manner. These statements should simply explain how the other person's words or actions make you feel and should not be any sort of personal attack. Be clear in your mind that it is all right to tell others how you feel and that it is OK to have negative emotions—it's a part of being human, and these emotions can be dealt with properly.

Review your emotional state daily

Complete a review of your negative feelings and emotions each day. What happened during the day? Did someone say something that made you angry or upset? Did something happen that left you feeling uncomfortable or saddened? Do you have an ongoing situation in life that is not easily resolved? Observe it, own it, and when you can, let it go, so it will have no further power over you.

As I return to my story here, I understood the mechanics of the problem, but I needed a method to resolve the tension and break this continuous cycle. My search took me on the two different paths that would bring me healing: one focused on the emotional cause of the tension, while the other dealt with the physical tension itself. My thoughts became preoc-cupied with these ideas, and I reread Dr. Sarno's book several times. So what did I have here? What did I need to do? There seemed to be two components: the physical tension and the negative emotions.

After I understood that my own mind was creating this tension, I knew that I needed a method to change the tension condition in my back and knees, so I created a relaxation technique that I call Total Muscular Release (TMR). This is not an exercise to be done once; it should become an important part of your daily routine to keep your tension and pain at bay.

Physical Tension

Total Muscular Release

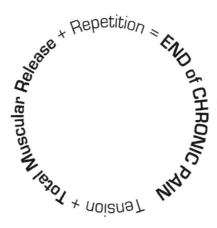

After twenty years, my lower-back muscles were a very stubborn case, indeed. While I was lying down, I had trouble even releasing my lower-back muscles at first. I saw this tension as my target, and I planned a physical change to my body to release my pain. It takes coordination between the mind and the back to take control of the muscles: flattening them out, letting them drop down to the floor, and keeping them that way. It was such a foreign state for my muscles to be in that I wasn't sure if they really were fully released. When I first started letting go of these muscles, they seemed to heat up that part of my lower back, and even though I still had pain, I could feel that there was something different about it. I knew it was the beginning of a very big change for me.

I practiced Total Muscular Release as many times a day as I could. Before I got out of bed in the morning, I began to let my low-back muscles go. Surprisingly, once I was aware of it, I realized that my lower-back muscles were just as tight while I was sleeping as when I was awake. I would make time, if only a few minutes here and there, for TMR. I wanted to break that vice-like lock that was holding my lower-back muscles so tight and keeping them in pain. At the end of the first day, I did not feel any better, though I would say that my lower back felt a little different. It is hard to describe, but I guess I could say I had an awareness of those muscles, which I'd never really had before. In fact, I'd never purposefully relaxed my lower-back muscles before, and that was genesis of this TMR process. *I could control these muscles—wow!*

As I continued, I found that my low-back muscles were a bit aggravated, and the whole area seemed warm and sort of full of little pains. I wondered if maybe this muscular release was *hurting* me somehow. Then I stopped to think, *How could releasing my own muscles hurt me?* I let go of that thought, and I continued on. I persevered, staying vigilant to the state of my lower back, and tried to not let a minute go by without thinking, *Are you letting your muscles relax? Are you breaking that grip of tension?* In time it became clear to me that the warming I was feeling in my muscles was obviously the reaction of those muscles receiving the oxygen they had been starved for all those years.

A couple of days had gone by, and I was not seeing the results that I had hoped for, and I started to become discouraged. I wondered if I was barking up the wrong tree and feared my approach was not enough to change my physical situation. I began to think that maybe this was a crazy idea and that I really couldn't end the suffering just by controlling the tension in my back, but echoing in my head were the words of doctors and chiropractors I had seen for years: "Your low-back muscles are so tight." Indeed, tight muscles were the cause of my chronic pain, and overcoming those constricted muscles was going to be the solution that would resolve my pain. Perhaps I was wasting my time, and I would never get rid of this pain, but did it hurt to keep trying? As I gave this TMR method more time, I discovered an interesting thing: my lower back had a series of contracted muscles that were part of my tension problem. During my TMR practice, I felt distinctive sets of different muscles that were released in a particular order. The first set was at the very center near the spine, the second further out, and the third on the very outside. I really didn't know the names of those muscles, and it didn't matter as long as I could release them at will. In truth, alleviating the tension was the only thing that ever worked for me.

Around the third day of consistently applying Total Muscular Release (I mean really, really keeping it at the top of my mind), letting those muscles drop, letting them release completely, I started to feel some relief. I honestly could not remember the last time that I felt no back pain. It wasn't all the time, but often after a TMR session, I would realize that *I have no back pain.* After I had that thought, I would begin to feel the muscles tightening up again, whether in minutes or hours. At that point, though, I perceived my back pain in a way I never had before; I now knew that I could just release the muscles, the contraction would disappear, and the pain would go away. It was a real moment of crystal-like clarity for me when I realized I had the power to actually control my muscles. I could manage it, and I could make my pain go away, essentially on command. Yes, I could do that!

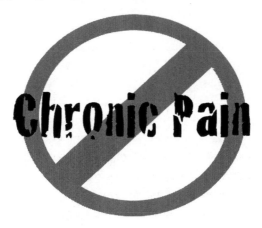

Since that time, my perception of why my life had been the way it was and what it might be like in the future has changed so dramatically. I am saying this without the slightest hyperbole. At that moment in time, everything changed for me, and I knew that this lower-back pain that had preyed upon me for all those years would eventually be gone—or at the very least, I could make it go away if it tried to return. I thought about the many people I've known who were absolute prisoners to their chronic pain. Some people were bedridden or essentially lived on the couch in their living rooms because they had so much pain they could not even get up to go to bed. Could TMR help them too?

Maybe you're thinking, *Could this be it? Can taking control of my target muscles and relaxing them on cue be the solution?* Well, if you are like me, once you master the skill you will start to be in control of your pain.

After a while, I realized that I could practice Total Muscular Release anywhere, and I did. Sitting at the dinner table, working on my computer, sitting in the car in traffic, walking into the office, or standing in an elevator—everywhere I went, I was relaxing my lower-back muscles.

One of my first chiropractors in Maryland told me that I should pull in my abdominal muscles while standing at the sink brushing my teeth or washing my face. I think he saw how unstable I was as I tried to get to a sitting or standing position, and this was his best advice. He was a very good chiropractor and got me up and going again after several devastating LBP crisis events. He certainly was trying to keep me from further pain, and it was probably the right advice for me in that state at the time. But everything I've learned since then tells me that pulling in muscles, holding muscles, and contracting muscles is the worst thing you could do when suffering from chronic tension pain. I think his instinct was right for me at the time, but in the long run, it made it worse and did not cure my pain.

The day I realized I was really able to mitigate my back pain made me even more determined to keep my back in a state of Total Muscular Release. I imagine I was fairly distracted during those days, as I kept checking in with all the muscles of my lower back and relaxing them, releasing them, and letting them go. It is difficult for other people to see your pain, but they can tell when your mood elevates, and that is the first thing my husband noticed about me. I hadn't told him what I was doing with

TMR, so he had no idea that anything was different with me or in the way I was feeling. One day shortly after my low-back pain was subsiding, he looked at me and said in a very upbeat way, "Wow, whatever you're doing, it has really done a lot for your mood!" That was an eye-opener for me, because I never saw myself as having a down mood. I guess my mood changed by degree along with my pain. Chronic pain year after year takes a lot out of you, and it affects your personality and the way you are perceived by others. TMR has given me so many things to be thankful for, and a happy mood was just another one of those gifts.

If you are trying Total Muscular Release for the first time, you may want to take a couple of days for yourself—maybe on a weekend, if you can spare the time—to practice the steps repeatedly. Being distracted will make it difficult to completely relax the target muscles and keep them that way. Having some time at the beginning may speed up the process and bring a faster end to the cycle of your chronic back-neck-shoulder pain. If you don't have a couple of days to dedicate to TMR, just keep working at it when you have time, and eventually you will find that you will be able to do it with ease.

Day 1	Chronic Back Pain
Day 3	Pain, but Changing
Day 5	Somewhat Lessened
Day 7	Pain-Free Blocks of Time
Day 10	No More Chronic Pain

Progression of Back Pain Relief.

My lower-back pain, the back pain I had ceaselessly for so many years, was gone about ten days after I started Total Muscular Release. It was clear to me during that period that I was getting a little better each day. I'd hoped against hope that TMR was going to bring me total relief, but I had no reason to believe it would. After being disappointed by doctor after doctor, I had little faith that this method would cure my chronic low-back pain in ten days. But if my pain could be reduced even by just 50 percent, I would be thrilled. Then one morning, I woke up and thought, *Hmmm, I'm lying here without back pain just after waking. Weird! I cannot remember the last time that happened.* I sat up in bed, checking in with my back, but there was no pain. I started to get out of bed gingerly, as always, expecting the familiar twinge that ran across my lower back for so many years, but still there was no pain. I walked around the room and down the hall—still no pain. *No way!* I thought. I truly cannot describe my elation when I realized that TMR was working for me. Only people who have suffered from chronic pain can understand what a joyous moment that would be. Of course, I had doubts and thought it may be a fluke.

I walked around a bit and realized that, for the first time in a very long time, I had *no* lower-back pain! I could not believe that this set of simple relaxation exercises and some emotional awareness could cause this amazing result so quickly and easily. I wanted to believe that this was the cure I had been waiting for all these years, but it was hard to trust it and know for sure that this was verifiably *it*. After all, I had been disappointed so many times before.

TMR continued to keep my lower back healthy and pain-free and made me feel more relaxed emotionally than I had been in years. I certainly was happier, because I was relieved of the burden of chronic pain. For the first time in years, I knew I would have no low-back pain from the time I woke in the morning to the time I went to bed. This brought an end to the chronic pain, and I felt as though an enormous weight had been lifted from my body and mind.

No longer being in the grip of chronic back pain was wonderful for sure, but I had a new target in mind, and that was my knees. Knee pain had been with me consistently for about three years, and I believed that the pain was the beginning of arthritis onset. We are constantly told that this is what to expect when we hit our fifties. Some of my family members had had knee pain in the past, which they attributed to arthritis, so I thought I had arthritis too. The pain was worst when I used the stairs. Sometimes going up was more painful, sometimes going down, and there did not seem to be any rhyme or reason to it. Some mornings I would get out of bed and have no knee pain at all, and other days I was in agony with every step all day long.

I enjoy the old German-built house that we have in Cincinnati, Ohio, but I was falling out of love with it with each passing laundry day. Carrying baskets of laundry up and down two flights of stairs with my knees complaining the whole way was getting old quickly. When I was a kid, we lived in a nice Cape Cod– style house with two sets of stairs, and I have pretty much always lived in houses with stairs since, and never had a problem with it, but I was beginning to think I would need to move to a one-level home in the not-too-distant future. Pain avoidance had me mentally planning all of the tasks I had to do on another floor so that I could reduce the amount of trips I had to make up and down the stairs. I knew it was a little crazy to have these thoughts, but that was how life was, and I learned to adjust to it. The company where I work is on the seventh floor of an office building, and before I had knee pain, I regularly walked up and down those flights for a quick workout, but after my knee pain began I would only use the elevator. I would see other people heading to the stairwell to walk down at the end of the day and think how I couldn't do that anymore. Sometimes there were scheduled fire drills in the building, and we would have to walk all the way downstairs and out to the street. It was a painful exercise, and I remember thinking, *What if it was a real emergency and I needed to run down the stairs?* Pain makes you think differently about many situations in life.

I wanted to believe that the TMR approach would be successful in relieving me of knee pain, but I had real doubts because I had this notion of arthritis. How could I get rid of my arthritis with TMR? Just the idea of being able to relax my knees seemed like it was going to be difficult. The knees—whether they are straight, slightly bent, or fully articulated—have active tendons and ligaments. The knee has many different parts—ligaments, tendons, cartilage, menisci, muscles, and bones—making it a very complex joint. It did not seem possible to be able to isolate the muscles of the knee joint for Total Muscular Release.

2 Weeks	Chronic Knee Pain
3 Weeks	Knee Pain, but Changing
4 Weeks	Knee Pain Lessened
5 Weeks	Pain-Free Blocks of Time
6 Weeks	Knees Pain-Free

Progression of Knee Pain Relief.

I approached the knee pain with TMR in the same way I had for my back pain and included targeting my knees along with my back. It took about four weeks from the time that I overcame my lower-back pain to completely resolve my knee pain. Wow, my knee pain was gone—I could run again, I could hike, I could walk up and down stairs without the dread of hurting; I was ecstatic! It appears there was no arthritis after all. When reflecting on the course of the resolution of my back and knee tension, I have come to understand that the knee pain was most likely caused by the condition created by the lower-back tension. It is clear to me that I needed to resolve the lower-back issues before the pain in my knees could be addressed. I remember someone telling me that the core muscles included all of the muscu-lature from the shoulders down to the knees, and now I've seen that it is all connected it in a very meaningful way. Please keep in mind that, if you are someone with multiple areas of pain, like me, you may need to work out one area of tension before another area can be resolved. Clearly many of these things are connected, both literally and figuratively.

While I was developing the TMR method I found a resolution to rest-less leg syndrome (RLS), which I suffered from on-and-off for many years. If you have RLS, or know someone who has tried to solve it, you know that it can be a sleep depriving, and maddening aliment to treat. I asked my doctor about it and she thought I might have a calcium deficiency. So, I began to take calcium, sometimes in the morning, and sometimes at night. After months of taking calcium and finding no relief I stopped taking it. I read about potassium, or a combination of calcium and potassium as a cure for RLS, and none of those minerals worked for me. Somewhere I read about magnesium for muscle problems. I started taking 300mg of magnesium before I went to sleep, and that did the trick. Apparently, all of that muscle contraction used up all the available magnesium in my body, which led to the RLS. Since my muscles are no longer in a contracted state all the time, I am not expending all of my magnesium daily, so I only take magnesium on days where I have worked my muscles strenuously.

If you're trying TMR and having some success, that's great, but now it's time to look at the other side of it, which is negative emotions.

Negative Emotions

A very important part of TMR is awareness of negative emotions and dealing with those emotions to the best of our ability. My understanding is that my negative emotions cause the autonomic nervous system to create tension in my body. That being said, I took to dealing with my emotions, which really just consisted of reviewing my emotional life each day. No one teaches us this skill and that's a shame, because not keeping tabs on our emotions can wreak havoc on the body. It certainly did in my experience. Sometimes I would do this in the morning and sometimes at the end of the day, but I would just walk through an inventory of my feelings; what was going on in my personal life, work life, and the world; and my immediate and long-term concerns. I would run through this inventory before or after I completed the relaxation portion of TMR. Just the act of identifying, reviewing, owning, and evaluating my negative emotions gave me a sense of peace and reduced the tension in my body. I didn't try to fix all the situations and problems in my life. I just took the time to look at what was going on, gave it some thought, and moved on.

Try to incorporate this simple emotional-review exercise into your daily routine as a way of reducing your tension and pain. We will always have some negative emotions—we are human, and that seems to be part of our condition, but they don't have to rule our bodies and lives. If you can tame your emotions, you can relieve your tension and, ultimately, your chronic pain. These self-evaluating practices are the key to breaking the cycle of chronic pain. First break the muscle tension and then find a way to reduce negative emotions.

There are many types of negative emotions driven by various sources, such as external and internal sources, or they may be directed by our moods. Sometimes we don't know where these feelings come from, and we often don't give those emotions much thought; it's just the way we feel, and that's the way it is. It would be nice if we always understood why we feel the way we do, but if you don't, that's OK—just review it, own it, and move along. No one wants to think about negative emotions because they are unpleasant, and it's a lot more fun to think about happy feelings.

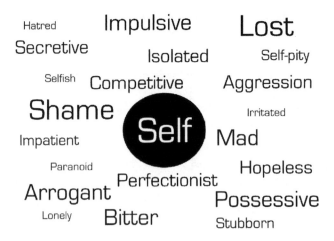

Below is a table that lists some of the negative feelings, internal and external, and the moods associated with them. This is by no means an exhaustive list, but it was added here to help the reader consider that negative emotions can be generated from various spheres of life and consciousness.

External	Internal	Mood
Jealousy	Nervousness	Depression
Annoyance	Uneasiness	Anxiety
Rage	Jitters	Worry
Displeasure	Anguish	Unhappiness
Exasperation	Regret	Grief
Fury	Panic	Desperation
Envy	Self-doubt	Sorrow
Hatred	Angst	Discouragement
Fear	Apprehension	Gloom
Indignation	Restlessness	Hopelessness

What emotions have you experienced recently? What emotions are you feeling right now? How intense are these feelings, and are you able to let some of them go? Maybe you can let them go maybe you cannot. If you feel during this examination of your feelings that you're having some serious conflicts, you may want to seek therapy to help you resolve these issues. Most people certainly have negative emotions from time to time—some more than others—and it is often based on our temperaments. Not all negative emotions are bad for us. Sometimes we need to find the emotional energy to correct a situation or get ourselves out of a spot that isn't in our best interest, and a negative emotion can be the charge that drives those necessary actions. Generally, negative emotions are just a reaction to certain stimuli or situations. If we can catch ourselves quickly enough when we are triggered by these events, we can stop, slow down, and disrupt those feelings so they don't transform into intense or entrenched emotions. It is not always easy to do, but it is a practice that we can aspire to if we put our minds to it. This type of negative emotion review can help you with your tension-based chronic pain, but is also a good idea for just about anyone.

The other way to sabotage negative emotions before they get a hold on us is to simply refuse to let that event, comment, situation, or whatever the issue may be have space in our minds. Just decide to let it roll off. For those emotions that have haunted us for some time, long-held grudges, slights, or hurts that drag on and on, let them go from your consciousness like a handful of feathers in the wind. Of course, letting go of painful emotions and feelings can be difficult, but it is harder to hold onto them and let them run your emotional life.

Stopping emotions from becoming negative at the start or letting go of long-held emotions is a great idea, but sometimes those things may not be possible. We will have emotions that are full of adverse energy; this is part of our human-ness. So what do we do about it? We must understand our emotions.

Knowing what's going on is most often better than not knowing what is going on. When I was in college, I took a train from Long Island to New York City each day. One summer there were several outages on my train line, and something happened at that time which has stayed with me these many years. The train stopped one day without warning, and we waited quite a while without hearing any announcement about what was happening. In short order the passengers were getting angry and grumbling, as it was hot and uncomfortable on the train. The conductor came through the car, and some of the passengers yelled at him about the delay. A week later the train stopped again, and this time an announcement was made immediately describing that a vehicle was stopped on the tracks ahead. There was some conversation but no one got mad, and no one yelled at the conductor because they were informed, and this made them feel they had some power in the situation. You can have some power in your situation, but you will have to take it.

When a child hears a noise in his or her room at night but is too afraid to get up to see what caused it, those thoughts loom large in their minds. The fear of the unknown is always so much scarier than the truth in this case. The child's fear causes them to tense up, and they can't fall asleep. It is always better to get out of bed, turn on the light, and take a look in the closet or under the bed to realize it wasn't really anything at all.

So get up, turn on the light in your mind, and take a look. At the beginning or end of each day, do an inventory of your negative emotions. What's been going on, whom did you have an unpleasant exchange with yesterday, and what future issues are you concerned about? Muse over these items in your head, and assign each a number on a simple scale of one to five. Think about the highest-rated issues. If you realize they aren't too important, they shouldn't have much of a hold over you, so see if you could consider dropping their ratings down even lower. For the items that you rated on the lower end of the scale, could you lower some of them even further? Can you drop them down so low that they fall off the list?

Do this exercise in your mind or on a grid like the one below each day. Try not to spend too much time on it or make it too complex, nor does it have to be an exhaustive list; this is a simple review of your current emotions, which will allow you to understand them and see if you can reduce their effect over your mind. If you're experiencing muscle tension due to negative emotions, these emotions are already taking up too much of your time and energy, so deprioritize them and spend your time on the things that are really important to you. The reason for this daily exercise is to reduce your negative emotions, reduce the tension, return blood flow to your target muscles, and end your pain.

You can use the chart below as a sample to track your negative emotions from week to week, or month to month if you choose.

Emotions Chart

Low: 1, Low–medium: 2, Medium: 3, Medium–high: 4, High: 5.

Negative emotion description	Current rating	New rating

This chart may be helpful to you when you get started on your negative emotion review, but after a while you may find that you can just walk through your list of negative emotions in your mind in. Hopefully in time, your list will get smaller, and this exercise will be accomplished in a couple of minutes per day. In thinking about my own recovery from chronic pain, I realize there were certain phases of activity as I moved through my healing. In the chapter Advanced TMR, I describe the three distinct phases of TMR, which I needed to pass through as I developed this method for breaking the pattern of chronic pain in my body.

■ ■ ■

Oxygen: The Cure

OXYGEN—IT FLOWS THROUGH our bodies (in and out of every cell of our bodies) every second of every day. An odorless, colorless gas in plentiful supply, it is free, and it surrounds us. Although we could not live a minute without oxygen, we rarely give it a thought. The task of breathing is done for us by our autonomic nervous system. The ANS has sensory and motor elements that govern inhalation, exhalation, heart rate, respiratory rate, blood pressure, digestive processes, body temperature, and other functions that allow it to maintain homeostasis (a state of relatively stable equilibrium between interdependent elements, as maintained by physiological processes). The ANS does a lot of the housekeeping, allowing us the freedom to perform other conscious tasks each day. Our breathing speeds up when the situation requires more oxygen, such as when we are running or exerting ourselves, and it slows down when we are at rest or sleeping. The ANS is, thankfully, a system that is generally on autopilot, and that is a very good thing.

Think for a moment what happens to us when we do have a momentary disruption to the flow of oxygen. Maybe you were in a swimming pool or at the ocean on a family vacation as a child, and while enjoying the water, you were suddenly unable to get to the surface for a couple of seconds or a wave knocked you down into the surf. What you experienced at the moment was instant discomfort and heaviness in your body—maybe a feeling of panic. After a first gasp underwater, you probably held your breath, which caused a muscle spasm of the larynx, and that was the beginning of hypoxemia (low oxygen in the blood).

When there is a lack of oxygen, our aerobic (oxygen-fueled) metabolism slows, and the body becomes acidotic, which will make us feel quite bad in very short order. All of these changes to our body's processes begin to happen in a matter of seconds, so you can imagine what would happen after days, weeks, months, and years of oxygen deprivation in *certain muscles*. If you are reading this book, you already know what it does to us—it delivers all-consuming, excruciating, and *chronic* pain.

If you've ever accidentally cut your finger on a knife or a piece of broken glass, then you know how painful that can be. It may take a moment to register with your brain that you have experienced an injury, and then you quickly feel that searing pain. The immediate reason for this pain is that you have experienced a decrease in blood flow to the site of the laceration. Those arteries, veins, and capillaries have been cut off from their source, and a pain message is quickly sent to the brain. Generally speaking, a lack of oxygen (ischemia) to any part of the body will bring pain.

Perhaps you were a runner in high school or college, or maybe you jogged at a local track or around your neighborhood for a good workout. Most people, whether they are runners or not, have experienced leg cramps, or what is sometimes called a charley horse. The muscles of the calf or elsewhere in the leg tighten up, and the pain comes on very quickly. Stretching out the cramping muscle or massaging it will often help to resolve most muscle cramps. Stretching and massage are activities that perform a certain function for the muscles, and that is to bring circulation, blood flow, and, of course, oxygen.

Could the pain be caused by lack of oxygen? When that thought first came to my mind, I was skeptical. Not once, ever, did a doctor even hint that my pain could be caused by a lack of oxygen. I was told many times by doctors that my back was in spasm, and the usual reason I was given was that my muscles were attempting to protect an injury. I later found that there was no injury except for the constant deprivation of oxygen to those muscles.

If you search on the Internet, you will find some web pages about back pain and lack of oxygen; this is not a new idea, but it seems to be a rare occurrence for doctors to discuss the role of oxygen in chronic pain.

Chronic pain can be intense and terrifying, so it's only natural that our minds assume we have a serious medical issue and that it couldn't be as simple as a lack of oxygen. Lack of oxygen was absolutely the cause of my pain for the better part of two decades. As soon as I resolved the muscle contraction, the oxygen began to flow again, and the pain was quickly gone—it was as simple as that.

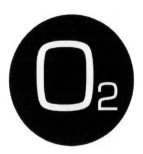

The NIH describes leg cramps as muscle spasms that occur when muscles are overused or injured. It goes on to describe things that may bring on muscle spasms, such as exercising while dehydrated or having low levels of minerals, such as potassium or calcium. The NIH goes on to say that spasms occur because the nerve that connects to a muscle is irritated and also reports that neck spasms in the cervical spine can be a sign of stress.

On its website (http://www.nlm.nih.gov/medlineplus/), the NIH notes that neck pain is muscle strain or tension and that everyday activities are to blame. A few of those activities include:

- bending over a desk for hours
- poor posture while watching TV or reading
- having your computer monitor positioned too high or too low
- sleeping in an uncomfortable position
- twisting and turning the neck in a jarring manner while exercising

So what is the cause of neck pain? Is it tension or activities?
And why would the NIH prescribe the following for tension?

- over-the-counter pain relievers, such as ibuprofen (Advil or Motrin IB) or acetaminophen (Tylenol)
- heat or ice applied to the painful area
- slow range-of-motion exercises
- gently massaging the sore or painful areas
- sleeping on a firm mattress without a pillow
- a special neck pillow
- a soft neck collar to relieve discomfort

NIH goes on to say that relaxation techniques and regular exercise to prevent stress and tension to the neck muscles can prevent or decrease neck pain.[12]

The message from NIH is somewhat confusing, and that is because it tries to lump all pain into the same category, which may be the reason that its advice is sort of all over the map. There are at least two kinds of pain, but for our purposes here, there are the temporary muscle aches, pains, and strains that happen when we overexert ourselves, and then there is chronic muscle pain, which is a very different type of pain. It is important to understand the distinction between these two ailments.

Temporary muscle aches are caused by some activity—some type of exertion that is unusual for that individual, such as running a marathon, taking a long canoe trip, a day of hiking, packing and moving, a new workout or exercise class, hours of gardening, and so on. This type of pain generally appears on the day after the activity, and it will often be resolved in two to three days, sometimes four to five days at most, as everyone's experience is a little different. In this scenario, there is no serious injury. Simply stated, some muscles were worked a little harder than usual, muscle fibers were torn, and they need time to heal for a few days.

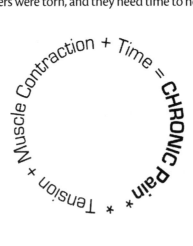

Muscle Contraction + Time = CHRONIC Pain * + Tension *

It is my experience that chronic back-muscle pain is a result of deprivation of oxygen (most likely caused by tension) to a certain set of muscles. This may start as an acute episode and is considered to be chronic after three months' time. The pain becomes chronic, because the muscles are under constant assault by ongoing tension, which continues to cause the muscles to contract, and the contraction continues to deprive the muscles of oxygen.

As long as the tension remains in those back, neck, or shoulder muscles, those areas will stay in a contracted state. When the muscles are forced into a contracted state, blood flow and oxygen will be restricted, and will result in pain. As long as this state continues, the pain will continue, and in time, it will become chronic. When you recognize this concept and accept that this is the root of your pain problem, you will understand that releasing tension is the first order of business in healing yourself and changing your life for the better.

NEGATIVE EMOTIONAL FEEDBACK LOOP

I've described the process of negative emotional tension causing the contraction of certain muscles, which reduces the flow of blood and oxygen and results in pain. However, there is a second, insidious segment of that route which I am calling a Negative Emotional Feedback Loop for this purpose. When someone begins to suffer chronic pain, that pain feeds back into the mind and the ANS, adding discomfort and stress to the existing roster of negative emotions. These additional negative emotions are then fed back down through the chronic pain path into the target muscles, along with the current set of negative emotional pain, which needless to say increases the pain burden.

As the chronic pain worsens from the additional negative emotional load, a new set of stressors begin to take hold, including emotional fear about the pain, uncertainty about the future, financial worries, anxiety, and potentially depression. With each new round of negative emotions and stress, the tension increases and there is a further lack of oxygen, which in turn brings even more pain.

This Negative Emotional Feedback Loop continues until exhaustion invariably sets in, and the sufferer can no longer fight it. The individual becomes incapacitated and unable to function in his or her life. People who find themselves in this weakened and debilitated state obviously did not get to that point overnight. This loop is a constant, self-feeding cycle that bombards them for months or years until they can no longer endure it. Over time, perfectly able, healthy people suffering in the Negative Emotional Feedback Loop can find themselves losing function until they are completely disabled by it.

The Negative Emotional Feedback Loop is illustrated in the panels below:

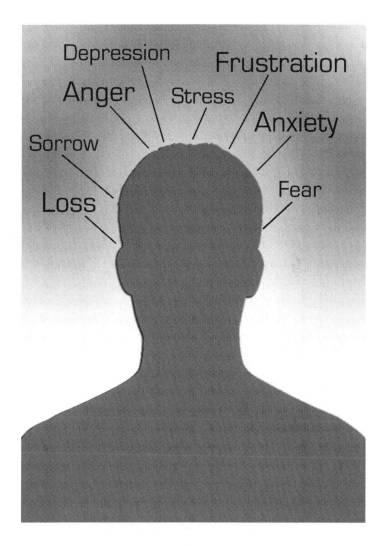

1. Negative emotions increase.

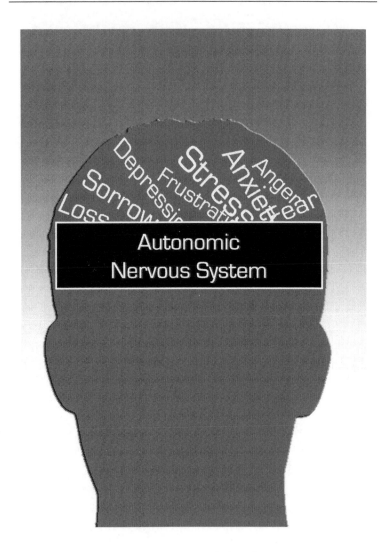

2. Negative emotions can overwhelm the autonomic nervous system.

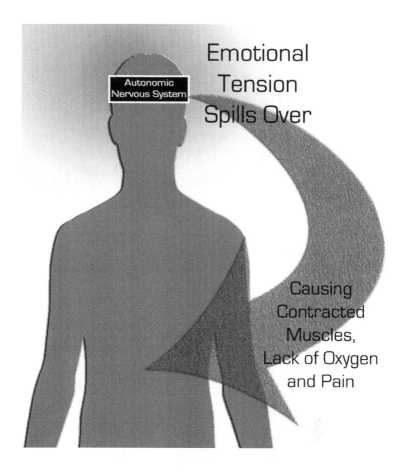

Emotional Tension Spills Over

Autonomic Nervous System

Causing Contracted Muscles, Lack of Oxygen and Pain

3. The emotional energy spills over and is displaced in the body as tension and muscle contraction. The muscle contraction causes a lack of blood flow and oxygen, resulting in pain.

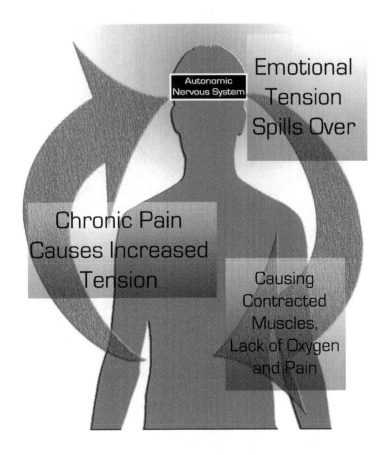

4. The pain experienced causes more stress on the autonomic nervous system, which continues the cycle with further muscle contraction, lack of oxygen, and pain.

Breaking this cycle is the first step to healing chronic tension-based pain. Everyone is different, and if tension is not the only cause of your back-neck-shoulder pain, and you may need to seek remedies elsewhere.

If anyone had told me earlier that a lack of oxygen was the cause for my chronic pain, I would never have believed it, but truly that was the reason I suffered all of those years.

■ ■ ■

Emotions Run the Show

C OULD YOUR OWN emotions be creating the chronic pain that has had a hold over you for months or years? The concept may be difficult to accept at first, but when you take a look at the human nervous system, you see that all neurologic pathways stem from the head and mind.

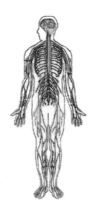

The brain acts as a director, making our bodies operate by sending different types of messages, hormones, electrical impulses, and other communications to various parts of the body. The nervous system sends chemicals in the form of neurotransmitters, while the brain's endocrine system and pituitary gland communicate with the heart, kidneys, liver, pancreas, and muscles through hormones. Our mind is the core of our emotional life, managing our many fleeting impulses of fear, love, joy, apprehension, worry, and pride mixed in with our memories, both positive and negative. The mind is the place where all of those important emotions commingle to help form us into unique and individual beings.

The mind is a stunning piece of biology that does a wonderful job of steering us around, creating hundreds of connections, building synapses at an amazing rate, and arriving at just the right set of decisions to keep us healthy, safe, and relatively happy. The mind is, without a doubt, the most impressive organ of the body and, strangely enough, one that we rarely give much thought about.

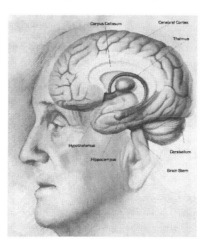

Diagram of human brain structures.

In the world in which we live, we suffer many assaults on our physical body, such as air pollution, contaminants in our food and water, and a myriad of other stressors. The brain also must deal with an endless array of troubles, concerns, and threats as it goes about the job of taking in sensory input from the outside world, using the information it has stored, and acting on that information for the good of the body and mind. This type of information processing happens at lightning speed and creates a great demand on our psyche, which is generally dealt with by the mind in an appropriate manner.

We know that animals in the wild suffer from stress as they try to survive, reproduce, avoid predators, etc. There are momentary periods of great stress when being chased by another animal or defending offspring or territory, which causes blood pressure to rise quickly and adrenaline to surge. When that threat has ceased, the animals' stress response drops, and they return to a state of normalcy.

The pattern of occasional extreme stress followed by a generally low level of stress most of the time was normal, and well tolerated by our ancestors in the past. Modern-day humans are generally rarely placed in a situation where they are truly in fear for their lives. The stress of contemporary life, however, can put human beings in an unnatural and constant state of chronic stress, although it is not life threatening situation. When thoughts ceaselessly continue to invade our consciousness and are never fully resolved, we are put at risk by this constant state of stress. When we have ceaseless thoughts about how we will make a living; worries about health, politics, climate change, families, jobs, the future; and a myriad of other concerns, it can hold us in a chronic state of stress.

Chronic emotional stress is not just bad for you but can also lead to crippling medical conditions, such as high blood pressure, increased heart rate, elevated levels of stress hormones, arteriosclerosis, clinical depression, and a compromised immune system. In combination, those conditions can bring illness, disease, a shortened life span, and chronic pain.

Our own emotions at the subconscious level can bring yet another layer of stress to the mind, and sometimes our minds respond by taking that energy and farming it out to other parts of the body in the form of muscle tension. Like many problems in life, this tension starts out small—so small that it may be imperceptible to us—and we may not even notice it at first. Eventually the pain rises to a level at which we are very aware of it, and we may try to ignore for a while, but ultimately we seek to resolve it.

The human body desires to keep us in a state of homeostasis, so it finds ways to cope and compensate to make our bodies work for us, until the demand becomes too great. At that point the body is in a vulnerable state, and when we may make just one more demand on those stressed muscles we can suddenly find ourselves in severe pain. The sufferer may have an acute attack of pain, and say that suddenly his or her back "went out," but in truth, there is no major damage and no bones broken; it's simply that those constricted muscles can no longer operate with a lack of oxygen, and that can cause a frightening amount of pain even under normal physical stress. These events are often short-lived because we treat the pain with rest, drugs, exercise, stretching, or some sort of therapy that brings those muscles enough oxygen to stop the pain. The pain goes away, and we call ourselves cured, until the next time. If our attempts at a cure do not bring enough oxygen to those starved muscles, we continue to have pain and eventually the pain will become chronic.

Tension is a feeling of nervousness that makes us unable to relax. In small doses, tension can be a helpful warning sign that something is not right, and when we feel it, we should pay attention to avoid trouble down the road. The problems with tension arise when it becomes our constant state of being and that previously temporary state becomes our new normal. Tension left unchecked will eventually lead us to issues with our health and may potentially result in chronic pain. We diligently attempt to find a solution from doctors, therapists, and through many other sources, but the underlying issue is still there. At some point, that initial urgency to find a cure for the pain may be replaced with a feeling of resignation; we give up, and we learn to live with the pain day in and day out. We look for pain *management* and forget about finding a cure.

This is where TMR comes in. When we have met a crisis point in our bodies, and pain, stress, and emotional discord are present, we must act. TMR can help us manage all of these things.

It certainly would be wonderful if we could all live peaceful, trouble-free, utopian lives in which we had no stress and our emotions never got the better of us, but that is an unlikely scenario for most of us. So what can we do? We need to recognize, observe, and own up to our stressors and learn how to manage our negative emotional stress effectively. Below you will find some practices to help you accomplish this.

SIX STEPS TO EMOTIONAL BALANCE:

1. Treat your emotions like any other part of your body. You brush your teeth, exercise, and eat the right foods to keep yourself healthy, so spend some time recognizing and understanding your negative emotions. Review them every day

to check in with what is bothering you: how much do these feeling bother you, and why? Explore what you can do to change a troublesome situation in your life, or find a strategy to reduce its importance in your emotional being.

2. Be honest with yourself about your emotions, which is not always easy to do. Instead of thinking about an emotion you are having and telling yourself that it really doesn't bother you, take some time to think about its true significance. Maybe the issue that you have been swatting away all these years is not just an annoying little gnat but more of a bear in your psyche. If you find that you have emotions you cannot get a handle on, seek out professional advice to help you manage it properly.

3. When you find that you are able, let go of difficult or painful emotions from the past. That is often easier said than done because we can, at times, carry a lot of emotional baggage around, even though it may no longer have any real significant meaning for us present day. Sometimes these are just old emotional habits that we repeat, which our minds continue to harbor because our brain likes to keep things. It may just be that we haven't given ourselves permission to let go of that hurt, grudge, or emotion, so it continues to have power over us. If these emotions are no longer serving a purpose for us, we should try to find a way to let them go.

4. If you find that you cannot let go of certain emotions, simply make it something you acknowledge, and review it again at another time.

5. Give yourself some time to quiet your mind by practicing meditation, deep-breathing exercises, creative visualization, prayer, or any contemplative exercise that is most relaxing to you. Taking some time to stop and slow your racing thoughts can be a peaceful retreat during your daily routine and is a great way to start or end your day.

6. Try to do some little kindnesses for yourself each day, such as giving yourself a massage or dry-body brushing, taking a long bath, eating healthy, getting plenty of rest, exercising, and understanding when you have done enough and it's time to rest. It never hurts to do some small kindness for someone else either, and that can make everyone feel good.

Completing these six practices will not completely remove tension from your life, but it may help to put you in a better emotional frame of mind and put you in touch with what is going on with you emotionally. Reducing the load of negative emotional energy can reduce the potential of tension in the body and guard against tension-related pain and chronic muscular pain. Coupling these mindful practices with TMR can help you feel relaxed and in control of your body and mind. It is no wonder, in these hectic lives that we lead, that we lose touch with our true emotional core. Our emotions can rule us, or we can seek to fully understand our emotional energy and make peace with it and ourselves.

■ ■ ■

Advanced TMR

WHEN I STARTED out on this TMR journey, I didn't know exactly what I was doing—it didn't even have a name yet—but it was clear to me that something important was happening from the start. As I found my way, I enhanced my muscle-release and negative-emotion-review practices and fine-tuned them to figure out what worked best for me. In this chapter, I'll provide further exercises you can follow to get the most out of TMR. Try the exercises listed here and you may want to change the approach slightly to find what is more effective for you.

Three Phases of Total Muscular Release

Phase 1 - IMMERSION

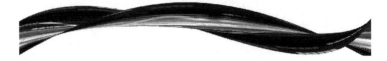

Starting TMR is a simple process but it will require practice to do it correctly, and get the best effect. If it doesn't work for you right away, please don't get discouraged. This is something that is completely within your ability, and it is a skill you can master. It took several days of practice for me to feel any change at all, and weeks before I had resolution. It may take a month or more for you to feel relief, which is fine; just keep working at it.

Begin by standing or sitting up, and reaching with your hands (if you are able to easily do so), touch the place(s) on your back, neck, or shoulders where you feel the muscle tightness. Maybe it is very obvious where the tightness is, or maybe your tension is at a lower level, so you can only feel the general area of tension. Think back to your doctor, chiropractor, masseuse, or other practitioner appointment in which they may have remarked about the tightness of your muscles. Where exactly are those muscles on your body? Can you feel them with your fingers and hands? If you are not able to feel them immediately, just focus with your mind on areas where you feel the tension and pain. Once you have identified your target muscles, you are ready to begin TMR.

TARGET MUSCLES

This portion of the TMR practice is the most important section and it was the beginning of my cure. Start by lying down on your bed, couch, or yoga mat (or wherever is the most comfortable place for you), and with your mind, calmly focus on those target muscles. I found that a yoga mat on a carpeted floor gave me a good, solid space to release my muscle down to while still being comfortable enough, but choose whatever surface feels best for you. Visualize where those tense muscles are located on your body. Close your eyes, take a deep breath in, and exhale all of the air out of your lungs. Begin to let those tense muscles in your back, shoulder, or neck fully release; let go of them, and let them drop downward. Feel those muscles releasing and easing a bit from each other and your body a little bit. The muscles will begin to sort of flatten out and feel a little warmer. You can adjust the position of your body slightly in place by rolling, rocking a tiny bit from the right to the left, and then easing back into a relaxed position, as you feel those muscles starting to smooth out. Adjust your body enough to give the muscles a little more room to expand and relax out fully. You can gently pull each arm across your body in turn to make sure you are giving your back and shoulders plenty of space on the surface to release.

Imagine that those troubled muscles are dropping to the floor, being completely calmed, warmed, softened, and allowing that entire section of your body to feel completely relaxed and free. At this point you hopefully are feeling quite flexible and serene. As you start to feel more at peace, the target muscles may start to feel a little warmer and your breathing may slow down a bit, which will help you feel more restful.

The ability to isolate a muscle or small set of muscles and completely relax them is not something that is generally taught in our culture. It requires a new kind of coordination, which you must develop. The direct connection between the brain and those muscles must be reestablished, and that contact must be kept open for you to continue to control those muscles and stop the pain. Once upon a time, maybe what seems like a long time ago, you had this open connection with your mind and those muscles, and there was no contraction or pain. When you were a child, you never gave muscle tension a thought, but you can make that easy, natural connection again.

Practicing these relaxation exercises will allow for that effortless, relaxed control that you had in the past. Continue to move into deep-muscle relaxation by dropping muscles down toward the surface you are lying on and adding the surrounding muscles as well. Again, your body will fight this because it is so used to being in a state of tension. This is not necessarily an easy thing to do—otherwise everyone would be able to do this without effort. Like any new thing that you take on in life, the start is very difficult, but with consistent practice, you'll get the hang of it and will be able to do it easily.

After ten to fifteen minutes of TMR, stop, take a break if you choose, and move on to something else for a while. If you feel that it is helping you at that time, continue to work on your release, and allow yourself to move into an even more relaxed state. It is normal to not feel any results at first, so don't worry, and try not to stress about it. I didn't feel much of anything for the first few days. In this early TMR pursuit, you are waking your target muscles up and telling them the old way is done, and it is time to change the way your body and mind interact. You are working to reduce the tension in your body, not increase it, so just relax and return to your practice later. TMR may come to you easily, or you may need to put more time into the method. You are at the beginning of a new way of being in your body, and following a course that will undoubtedly take some time and effort.

Whenever you have a few minutes to spare, stop and take a quick TMR break. Lie down, take a few deep breaths in and out, and begin to fully release your target muscles. Release, relax. Release, relax. Repeat this gentle muscle unwinding slowly and with purpose. The more times you practice TMR, the more quickly it will become second nature. Before you know it, you'll be feeling your target muscles relaxing in just minutes after you begin, and in time, you will be able to release those muscles in seconds. Even if you have a busy life or a chaotic household that puts a lot of demands on your time, be sure to find a way to grab those ten to fifteen minutes a few times a day.

Vanquishing chronic pain can seem like a herculean effort, but think of it more like an Olympic event in which you want to compete in the near future. You have the knowledge, you have all the equipment you need, and you have a motivated coach who has your best interest at heart—you. Take your TMR practice as seriously as you have taken any other effort you have expended to find a solution to your chronic pain. Train to eliminate your pain!

You are worth the time and effort that you need to make yourself well. Your pain is real and it can be devastating to the quality of your life. The physical pain caused by muscle contraction and the lack of oxygen is a physical aliment, and it deserves to be resolved. At the very least, try to practice TMR twice a day—when you first wake up and before you go to sleep, for instance—but try to get in as many sessions as are comfortable for you at the beginning. An important part of TMR is breaking those bad muscle habits that are very much ingrained in your body and mind. The more you can break that grip of tension the better off you will be. That kind of dramatic seed-change takes effort and time.

Curing chronic pain with TMR is sort of like taking on a flexibility task that you are not currently able to do, such as a handstand or a split. What you need is a plan for how to achieve your goal, and then you need to work the plan. If you were training yourself to do a split but you rarely practiced the skills necessary, it would take you a long time to be successful at it. The practice of TMR is very much the same in that regard.

It may be helpful to reflect on what is really going on in your body when you first begin to practice TMR. You are in a *battle* between your conscious and subconscious minds—maybe this is the first time in your life that you have considered the possibility of such a conflict. For the first time, your conscious mind is talking openly with your subconscious mind about the tension in your body. You undoubtedly have never had this type of conversation with yourself before, because you wouldn't imagine that such a dialog would be necessary. If you have out-of-control muscular tension that is causing you pain, I assure you that such discussions are crucial to breaking your chronic pain cycle.

Performing TMR is like a conversation in which your conscious mind says, "Muscles, you may *not* be tight; you *will* relax; you *will* let go and be at peace," while your subconscious mind says, "Wait, hold on...I have been dumping all this emotional energy into these muscles for a long time; I don't want to stop now, and I don't know what else to do." That is a battle you have been losing while you experienced chronic pain, but now you will turn things around, and believe it or not, you will come to a peaceful accord with your subconscious mind. I am using the word *battle* in this context to describe a conflict, but I don't want readers to feel they are at war with themselves, although when we are in the throes of a chronic pain episode, it can feel that we are at odds with our own bodies. Overcoming this situation can only happen if a win-win resolution is found between the mind and the body. We are working to gain control of the physical side of chronic pain, and we are also managing the psychological side of the issue. The more comfortable we feel having this conversation with ourselves, the more quickly we can find relief.

When I was at my most tense before I discovered TMR, I would describe myself as "holding myself up above the mattress." Of course I wasn't levitating above my bed, but my back and shoulder tension was so extreme, my muscles so tense, that it felt like I was being held up in the air by it. That type of severe tension is very unnatural, unhealthy, and extremely harmful to the body. Thankfully, these days I can release every muscle in my back and trunk without thought. It just took practice, and it was well worth the time invested.

TMR may sound somewhat nebulous when reading it for the first time, but just continue to work with it. Being able to relax any of the muscles in our body is normal, and it is something we should all be able to do easily. When we lose the ability to naturally release our muscles, we need to find a way to regain that function. Your mind created the tension in those muscles, and it can also let go of it, but only if we consciously make it happen. You may find that the muscles you've targeted will begin to tighten back up within a few minutes, which is to be expected, because your body has been in that contracted state for such a long time. Do not worry; just continue to let the target muscles relax, slacken, let go, and drop down. You are in the process of breaking patterns that your body has been holding onto, and it will resist this new initiative. Change can be arduous, but finding a way to live without chronic pain is certainly worth your efforts. Have patience with yourself as you begin, knowing that you will get better at TMR, and it will get easier for you with time.

Breathe into Your Muscles

BREATHING

In yoga and Pilates practices, teachers will often suggest that students "breathe into" their calves, arms, side, back, or whatever body part they may be working on during the executed pose. When I first heard that phrase, I have to admit that it did not make any sense to me. How exactly would I be able to breathe into my thighs? It just sounded strange. I eventually came to understand that what they really meant was that we were to *focus* on the muscles in that part of the body while fully exhaling. This is a technique that works very well with TMR. Simply exhale normally, or a little more deeply if you prefer, and place your complete focus on relaxing that part of the body.

Incorporate this simple breathing technique into your TMR practice each day as you relax your target neck, shoulder, or back muscles, exhaling out in a long, slow manner as the muscle completely relaxes. TMR is the performance of gentle muscle relaxation, so we are not stretching or physically elongating any muscles as one might do in yoga or Pilates. These muscles do not need to be worked out; they have been worked long and hard enough already. In TMR, we want these muscles released with a sensation of warmth and peacefulness. You'll find that breathing into your muscles sort of hyper-focuses your energy into relaxing your target muscles. This breathing process should be done in a calm, relaxing manner, and there is no need to exhale dramatically. You are trying to release the tension in your body, and if you are doing a lot of exaggerated breathing action it will make you tense up, which will not help you reach a state of complete TMR. Placing all of your energy into target muscle relaxation, breathing into the muscle, and using self-talk to dispel tension and pain is a triple threat against chronic muscle tension.

If you don't see results right away, don't be discouraged, and do not quit. You have the ability to take back the control of those contracted muscles that are causing your pain, but it may take some time. When you were a baby or a child, you most likely never suffered from chronic pain, because you had no tension and you had no pent-up emotions. If you were mad, you would yell, or maybe you threw a temper tantrum in the grocery store. If you felt sad or upset, you cried, and that tension created by your negative emotions was quickly dissipated. Expressing our negative emotions as they occur is an efficient system for dissipating negative emotional energy. This worked very well when we were young, but as we get older we begin to throttle our emotions, and that is where the trouble begins.

Once you are able to completely physically release those target muscles, you will most likely feel that they will attempt to return to their state of tension. This is muscle memory, which is similar to a rubber band that snaps back into its original shape. When I first began TMR, I wasn't really sure it was working, because although I could feel my muscles release during a TMR session, I found that the state was a short-lived one once I returned to my usual activities. I was pleased to find that eventually the relaxed state of my muscles became the permanent state, but it did take a while. You can implement a reset on those muscles, break that pattern of tension-contraction-lack of oxygen-pain, and help them find their new normal. In time you can overcome this muscle tension with your continuous, gentle TMR practice. When you feel that familiar muscle-tightening, simply stop it by letting the muscles release. Once you reach the point where you can successfully release your target muscles at will, even for short periods of time, you will have that learned that skill; then it's only a matter of time and persistence until you can completely break the pain cycle.

Continue this practice at least twice daily, and more often if you have the luxury of some extra time, so that you train your body to quickly and easily move the muscles into a relaxed state. Check in with your emotions on a daily basis to help lessen their impact on your mind and body. In my experience, it was the underlying emotions that I was not so aware of that may have been causing some of my tension and pain. When I really took the time to review all of my feelings and emotions, while continuing my TMR practice, I found that my muscle tension essentially disappeared.

Phase 2 - VIGILANCE

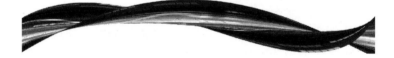

After you are able to release your target muscles on a reliable basis while lying down in a relaxed position, you'll begin to practice TMR in other positions wherever you are throughout the day. You will take your TMR practice to all the places where you sit, and stand, and go about your daily work, school, and home life. Relax your target muscles first thing in the morning when you wake up, as you sit up and prepare to get out of bed. Continue while you are standing at the bathroom sink brushing your teeth, drinking your coffee or tea at the breakfast table, sitting in the car in traffic, standing on the platform waiting for your train, standing in line at the grocery store, sitting in the stands at your child's soccer match—everywhere you go during your day. Proactively work on your muscle release in the many situations where muscular tension can begin to creep up on you.

Think of this as your new job; take it very seriously, and try to think of it as a healthy obsession. Your mission is to work to undo years and years of physical muscle memory. These patterns of tension dumping on your muscles by the autonomic nervous system are well ingrained, and need to be broken in order to stop the pain. This is no small effort that you are attempting here; it is absolutely a reprogramming of your mind and body. Breaking these bad mind-body habits takes the repeated application of new, positive habits, in addition to time and will. Use your resolve to rewire these major mind-body connections to realign your body and your health.

COMPLETE RELEASE WITH SELF-TALK

Hopefully, you have mastered TMR for your target muscle(s), and the next step is to work your entire body from head to toe. You had tension in a certain part of your body, but that doesn't mean that it won't find a foothold in some other part of the body. My experience has taught me that muscle tension could pop up in almost any part of my body, although for me it was generally in my back, lower body, and legs. It became clear to me that my body was hardwired to have this tension-dumping process occur, which required me to have a whole-body tune-up process to avoid any tension-pain issues in the future.

In this complete release practice you will perform this series of re-laxations with positive, directive self-talk. That might sound strange at first, but every action is born out of an idea, and these self-talk statements will tell your body what you want from it. Complete release with self-talk is a continuation of the conversation between the conscious and the subconscious minds. Try verbalizing your self-talk right out loud or just run through these phrases quietly in your mind while you work through each muscle group. During this whole-body practice, you may want to say something like, "I will *not* have any tension in my face, in my jaw, in my eyes, and in my brow," while you slowly relax all of the muscles in the face, around the eyes, in the forehead, and in the front of the head. You'll be sur-prised to discover how much tension is held in your face and head. Next, move on to the back of the head and say, "I will *not* have any tension in my head," while letting go of the scalp, ears, and back of the head. Say, "I will *not* have any tension in my neck" in a direct voice as you let the muscles around the back, front, and sides of the neck go slack.

One of the benefits I found after I started working with whole-body TMR was that the furrow in my brow began to relax. Naturally, I have a bit of an expression line in my brow, but what had been just a little line was becoming a crease as the years went by. I was unaware of it, but my tension and pain caused my brow to scrunch up most of the time. Indeed, chronic pain can cause a lot of grimacing. After I spent time focusing on relaxing my face, head and neck muscles, I discovered that I carried a lot of tension there, even though I had no pain in those areas. In addition to cur-ing my chronic pain, my whole-body TMR practice has taught me many things about my body, such as the facial tension mentioned above, or that a seated posture, which should be quite benign, causes a great amount of tension in my back and legs. I probably would have remained unaware of these things if I hadn't gone through this process.

We get so busy in life with the many demands, which are made on us by others and ourselves. The human body is so wonderful at coping with stress that it can be easy for us to lose touch with it, because somehow everything is still working for us. This chronic pain we experience is introduced by degree over time, as our body slowly loses its battle in trying to manage tension. When lose touch with what is going on with our bodies, we can find ourselves with chronic pain and other debilitating conditions. TMR can be a reset in many ways and can help us become knowledgeable about the way our bodies function.

Move down into your shoulders and say, "I will *not* have any pain in my shoulders." When I relax my shoulders, I think of it as though there is an oval around my upper shoulder area. I release each muscle in order from one shoulder, to the back, to the next shoulder, and around to the front again. Imagine that someone is sweeping a hand gently around your the entire shoulder structure until it is in a completely relaxed state.

Continue to work through your entire body, section by section, working down through the upper arms, the elbows, the lower arms, the wrists, the hands, and all the way to the ends of your fingertips. Continue your muscle relaxation using your mind, sliding down through the sides of the body. Take some time to loosen all of the muscles in the chest and abdomen, and be sure to breathe all the way out while you relax through the trunk of your body. The chest and the abdomen can be places of great tension for some people. Voice coaches often encourage their students to relax their chest, abdomen, and diaphragm to improve their singing and speaking voices. Try to spend some extra time in relaxing all of your abdominal and chest muscles.

If you are suffering with chronic back pain, you'll want to slowly move down through each section of the back. Start with the upper back just below the shoulders, down slowly through each section of the middle back, and into the lower back. Try to break each of these sections down into as many discrete releases as you are capable of identifying. There are over 300 pairs of muscles in the human back, so there is a lot of potential for muscle isolation. In my own TMR I found there were three separate sets of muscles in the lower back that had to be released in a natural order from the center outward. These muscles were absolutely key for me to find a way to break my tension and end my chronic pain.

Continue your TMR downward through the sacrum and the coccyx, isolate and release each hip separately, and then relax the entire pelvis. Finding a method to isolate parts of the pelvis was very challenging for me. It took me a while to get a fix on the muscles of the sacrum and the coccyx, but I now find this easy to do. I found that the muscles of the sacrum and coccyx acted as the glue that held my pelvis so tightly together, so discovering a way to relax them was imperative. The relaxation of each individual hip turned out to be a crucial step in removing tension from my pelvis, which I believe had contributed greatly to my pain. When the pelvis is too tight, movement is restricted in a manner that can bring pain. Maneuver your relaxation down through the thighs, knees, calves, and into the ankles, feet, and toes. While you work through your complete release, spend extra time working on your target muscles. Once you have run through this whole-body TMR process, your body should be in a relaxed state.

After completing the steps above, repeat these relaxation exercises in the same order again, but now say, "I will *not* have any pain in my face, jaw, eyes, or brow," etc., and again work down through your entire body as you did in the previous exercise. These tension and pain statements have been organized in a logical order like a line of dominoes. Knock down the tension in those muscles, and you will no longer have the contraction and lack of oxygen; then you should not have any pain. No tension, no pain. Try the self-talk phrases listed above at first so you can get used to the practice. After a while, you may want to create phrases that are more helpful or meaningful to you. If you use this technique correctly, you should feel at ease, be in a pleasant and relaxed state, and be ready to fall asleep. Sometimes I will run through this complete release self-talk process just to put myself in a pre-sleep state.

If this type of self-talking practice does not come easily to you at certain times, try not to stress about it. Perhaps you have a lot of things on your mind at the moment that may make it difficult for you to concentrate on your self-talk as you move through the exercises. Simply stop the exercise and pick it up later in the day, or at another time when you feel a little less distracted and better able to concentrate.

Continue the habit of complete release even if you do not have acute pain in that area, because you may find that it is helpful in discovering areas of tension that you were unaware of previously. If you can root out these tension areas, it will hopefully circumvent future muscle contraction, lack of oxygen, and pain episodes. Self-talk can be a difficult thing for many people to take on because it is new to them. Suddenly you are being asked to talk to yourself, but what should you say? Does this sort of thing make you seem a little crazy? The truth is we all talk to ourselves on a regular basis as we move through our daily lives. There is always a dialog going on in our minds about what we are doing and planning. Whether we're reassuring ourselves that things are going to be OK or giving ourselves a little pep talk before we try something new, we are performing a form of self-talk. During TMR we are conversing with our muscles and our subconscious mind to solve a problem.

All human endeavor starts with a thought or an idea. First we need to conjure an idea in our mind, and we have to believe it is viable, and then we can build it. Self-talk is a common way of working through issues, and it is something that should make you feel comfortable and relaxed. You know what you want from your body and your mind, so you need to ask for it. Stating clearly what your expectations are is the first step to making something happen. In this circumstance, you would be talking to your subconscious and telling it that you want it to stop creating tension in your body as you release your muscles at the same time. You will then tell your subconscious that you will not have any pain. It is not very easy to get the subconscious to reveal itself, as it operates in an undercover mode by nature, but by having this open dialogue with yourself, you can help to assure that your emotional life won't get away from you, as perhaps it did before. You are the only one who can have a successful conversation with your subconscious, so it is up to you to make the messages loud and clear.

Phase 3 - MAINTENANCE

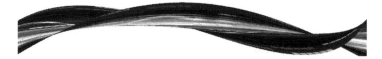

If you have successfully completed phases one and two and you are starting to have less tension and pain, or maybe you have no pain at all with your continued TMR practice, congratulations to you! You have now reached the final phase: maintenance. This third phase begins when you no longer have chronic pain, or are nearly pain-free, and you are ready to go on with life, knowing you have the tools to deal with tension in the future. At this point you may let your guard down just a bit, and you probably won't need to practice TMR as often as you did in the previous phases. Take some time to celebrate your achievement of breaking the cycle of chronic pain!

On a daily basis, continue to monitor your feelings and emotions when you have some time. Check in with yourself for a few minutes so that you can take a measure of any negative emotions brewing in the background. If there are some new or strong feelings there in your mind, you know exactly what to do about them: simply acknowledge them, own those feelings, understand that they are part of life, and then move on. Let those feelings go if you can, and if not, examine them at another time. Human beings have these emotions, and they always will, and there is no shame in it. Observing them and letting them go is the answer.

You'll want to practice TMR and complete release during the maintenance phase from time to time as a support to your mind-body health. This should be quite easy for you now, and you should be able to walk through the exercises without much thought. Sometimes you will find that your target muscles want to return to the state that they had been in for a long time, particularly during periods of greater life stress. This is just a temporary setback, which you can overcome by applying TMR to those muscles under tension. As soon as you feel that tightening, which you'll recognize immediately now, you will find comfort in knowing that you have the power to stop it, and simply let those muscles release.

Sometimes we go through stress in our relationships, or issues with health, finances, or other concerns. Those types of stressors can be a trigger for tension and pain, so be ready for it, and practice TMR before you start to feel the pain. If you are regularly checking in with your emotions, you probably already know that there are certain concerns that may be an issue for you. Continue TMR and the complete release exercises until you are through this current emotional episode. Stop and take a look at your calendar for the next week, and you may be able to identify these potentially volatile situations before they come up, such as a delicate work meeting or a visit from a difficult relative. If you can see a future episode that may introduce stress, be proactive and practice TMR before, during, and after the event.

ACTIVE TMR

This section includes information that is not necessary for successful TMR, but I have found it is helped me take my target muscle relaxation to another level. After having mastered the relaxation of target muscles in my entire body while lying down, and then following that effort by relaxing my target muscles while sitting or standing, I upped my game by using muscle relaxation in active physical states. My first steps in practicing active TMR were in relaxing my target muscles while walking around the house, while running errands around town, or while taking a walk around the block in my neighborhood. Active TMR was more challenging for me, as I had to put a lot of concentration into letting go of my target muscles, and I was not able to fully release them at the beginning consistently. Before I started I would do a quick check of my emotions to see if there was anything bothering me. Even if I did have some issues on my mind, I would find that just having that awareness relaxed me a bit.

I continued to practice TMR during activities such as fast walking, hiking, walking up and down stairs, jogging, yoga, and swimming. Eventually, I was able to reliably relax my target muscles during active TMR. Previously, I found that when I performed certain activities, they could sometimes be a trigger for muscle tension. Of course while we are active, certain muscle groups are contracting and releasing as necessary to operate. As I continued to relax my trigger muscles while I was active, I found that over time my target muscles were automatically in a relaxed state at the onset. My guess is that before I discovered TMR my target muscles were very tight during physical activities, although I was unaware of it at the time. Once I discovered that I could totally relax those muscles while I was jogging, or completing the yoga pose downward dog, a very physically active pose in which almost the entire body is engaged, I felt that I had reached a point where I really had total control of my tension. I now controlled the tension that had had total control of me for so long, and this is still amazing to me.

The end of years of low-back pain was a joyous relief, but the knowledge that I had the ability to overcome my pain by using my mind to break my tension made me even more at ease and confident.

I enjoyed my new found freedom from back pain, and this skill was empowering in nearly every area of my life. I didn't have to worry about some sudden pain incident that would stop me from working or doing what I wanted. This new ability removed so much of the dread I'd had from attempting normal activities like sitting in a chair, a seat in a car, or an airplane seat. I now could walk through a city, jog in the park, or hike up a mountain without fear that my pain would stop me. It allowed my life to become so much more fluid and effortless.

As I reflect on it, this was really a "Dorothy from *The Wizard of Oz*" moment for me in that I had the power to cure my pain all along, but of course I didn't have the knowledge. If I had only known about TMR practice, I wonder how different my life might have been. Would I have taken more risks, been more active, been more adventurous, had more confidence, been less distracted, and had more peace in my life? There is no way to know for sure, but living without chronic pain certainly would have been a much better way to live. I did seek medical care from professionals for decades, but none of them had the answer for me. In this case it seems that I was my own best professional.

"If wishes were fishes, we'd all cast nets."

- Frank Herbert

Do I wish I knew then what I know now? I'm sure you can guess that I dearly would have wanted the knowledge of TMR when I was first struck with LBP. I believed that chronic back, neck, and shoulder pain is just something that has to be managed, as many people do. I bought into the mantra of pain management as the only way to deal with chronic pain. Maybe this is what you have been told, and what you have always believed, but challenge yourself to think differently; live your life in a new way, and try another way of being. This is why it is so important to me that you, dear reader—and everyone suffering from neck-shoulder-back pain, or other chronic pain—get this message so that you can be free of chronic pain.

Chronic pain caused by muscle tension is not some crazy, in-your-head, imaginary pain; this is a real physical manifestation in the body due to stress, muscle contraction, and a lack of oxygen, and it is something that needs to be corrected from the inside. I cannot imagine that there is anything special or different about my chronic LBP, and I am sure that what worked for me will work for hundreds, thousands, and maybe millions of people around the world. It will, of course, only bring relief if people hear about it, have a willingness to try it, believe in it, and apply these simple principles.

Once there are more people who find some relief through this method, I am hopeful that we can start to have a dialog about tension-based pain, and the role the mind plays in this terrible affliction. The very worst that can happen as a result of practicing TMR is that readers will be a little more relaxed and, perhaps, be better in touch with their emotional life. I want all chronic pain sufferers to live that *better life* that I have finally found.

■ ■ ■

Current Research on Chronic Back-Pain

B ACK PAIN IS one of the most common physical ailments in the population of the world, and, therefore, it may also be one of the most studied of all physical conditions. A few simple searches of PubMed studies (online resources of more than 24 million citations for biomedical literature from MEDLINE, life science journals, and online books) alone yield the following results:

Search term	Number of studies
Low-back pain	22,545
Chronic low-back pain	3,925
Neck pain	7,962
Shoulder pain	5,549

In the section below, there are abstracts of recent reviews of clinical trials, which include hundreds of studies on tens of thousands of patients from around the world. The amount of time, money, and energy required to design, develop, execute, and review these clinical studies is a monumental effort, but sadly, the gains have been so few.

After all of this endeavor, there seems to be almost no consensus on the cause or cure of LBP or many other chronic conditions. This voluminous research has brought fairly little hope to the chronic back-pain sufferer. Some of the studies conflict with each other as to what causes chronic pain or what will heal it. Many studies draw little or no conclusion about what helps back pain in the short or long term. When I consider the poor state of the understanding of chronic pain and its cause and cure, I cannot help but think that they may be missing what may be right in front of them.

Note: the *italicized* text is added for emphasis.

Review of Scientific Research for the Treatment of Chronic Pain

Research has found that *chronic back pain* is a much more difficult problem, which often has strong *psychological overlay*, and that even *disc protrusions* detected on x-rays are often blamed; it is found that they *are very rarely responsible for the pain,* and *surgery is seldom successful* at alleviating it. The same study found that *treatments described as "heroic" ultimately fail* to help patients, may even be harmful, and should be avoided.[3] In a 2007 study, researchers concluded that *traction as a single treatment for LBP was probably not effective.*[4] Traction is not often prescribed these days, but it was the standard of care for back pain in decades past.

3 *Med Clin North Am* 98, no. 4 (2014): 777–789, doi:10.1016/j.mcna.2014.03.005, Patrick N(1), Emanski E(1), Knaub MA(2).

4 . *Bulletin of the World Health Organization* 81 (2003): 671–676, George Ehrlich, http://www.who.int/bulletin/volumes/81/9/Ehrlich.pdf.

A study concluded that *adverse psychosocial work conditions (high work demands) may contribute to the development of neck/shoulder symptoms through the mechanism of stress-induced, sustained muscular activation.*[5] Many chronic pain sufferers would agree that pain of the neck, and the shoulders are often caused by stressful work environments.

In a review of medications, a study found *insufficient evidence to identify any one medication as offering a clear overall net advantage* because of complex trade-offs between benefits and side effects.[6] Those who have tried multiple medications know that pain meds rarely bring long-term relief, and that side effects of these drugs are always a concern.

In a 2006 study review, medications with good evidence of short-term effectiveness for low-back pain are NSAIDs, acetaminophen, skeletal muscle relaxants (for acute low-back pain), and tricyclic antidepressants (for chronic low-back pain). Evidence is insufficient to identify one medication as offering a clear overall net advantage because of complex tradeoffs between benefits and harms. Individual patients are likely to differ in how they weigh potential benefits, harms, and costs of various medications.[7]

In a 1997 review, a study found that scientific evidence was limited for the efficacy of intervention for patients with low-back pain in

5 . "Traction for Low-Back Pain With or Without Sciatica," *Cochrane Database Syst Rev* 2 (2007), http://www.ncbi.nlm.nih.gov/pubmed/17443521.

6 . "Antidepressants for Nonspecific Low-Back Pain," *Cochrane Database Syst Rev* 1 (2008), doi:10.1002/14651858.CD001703.pub3.

7 . "Medications for Acute and Chronic Low-Back Pain: a Review of the Evidence for an American Pain Society/American College of Physicians Clinical Practice Guideline," *Ann Intern Med* 147, no. 7 (2007): 505–514, http://www.ncbi.nlm.nih.gov/pubmed/17909211.

terms of sickness absence rates or duration of sick leave. The authors formulated three main points from the review for the guidelines for occupational physicians:

- Bed rest should be limited or even avoided; normal activity should be continued as much as possible.
- If any conservative treatment for patients with acute low-back pain is considered, spinal manipulation is the best option.
- Antidepressants can be helpful for chronic low-back-pain patients.

The authors found promising results for exercise and education programs, especially for intensive programs in an occupational setting. However, those positive finding have not yet been confirmed in randomized clinical trials with sufficient statistical power and vocational outcome parameters.[8]

In a 2009 study, authors concluded that *there was insufficient* evidence to support the use of injection therapy in subacute and chronic low-back pain.[9] Many sufferers find no relief at all from injections but may be at risk of injury from the procedure.

A 2003 systematic review of randomized and/or double-blinded controlled trials concluded that muscle relaxants are effective in the management of nonspecific low-back pain, but the adverse effects require that they be used with caution. Trials are needed that evaluate

---

8 . "Vocational outcome of intervention for low-back pain," *Scand J Work Environ Health* 23, no. 3 (1997): 165–178, doi:10.5271/sjweh.195.

9 . "Injection therapy for subacute and chronic low-back pain: an updated Cochrane review," *Spine* 34, no. 1 (2009): 49–59, doi:10.1097/BRS.0b013e3181909558.

if muscle relaxants are more effective than analgesics or nonsteroidal anti-inflammatory drugs.[10]

A 2010 study reviewed thirty randomized trials (3,438 participants) and the authors found that, for patients with CLBP, there was moderate-quality evidence that operant (behavior modification) therapy is more effective than no treatment in the short term, and that *behavioral therapy is more effective than usual care for pain relief*, but they found that no specific type of behavioral therapy is more effective than another.[11]

In the research described above, tens of thousands of patients were studied by untold numbers of highly skilled researchers, doctors, nurses, clinicians, and other health-care providers in countries around the world. How is it possible, after decades in research, expending hundreds of millions of dollars, that we still cannot arrive at a cure for this devastating, chronic, global disability? Surely those involved must be greatly disappointed that decades of enormous effort have sadly yielded so little in terms of a cure for the millions of back-pain sufferers.

It may be that the current thinking in chronic-pain science causes researchers to continue to bark up the wrong tree, to use a well-worn expression. These lines of thinking force researchers to pursue directions that have not yielded answers and will most likely never take them down the path of finding the solution to the complex problems of LBP and CLBP. Persistently seeking a solution in the physical body, when physical pain may be just a symptom of the real problem, will most likely produce unsuccessful results in the future. It is difficult

---

10 . "Muscle relaxants for nonspecific low-back pain," *Cochrane Database Syst Rev* 2 (2003), http://www.ncbi.nlm.nih.gov/pubmed/12804507.

11 . "Behavioural treatment for chronic low-back pain," *Cochrane Database Syst Rev* 7 (2010), doi:10.1002/14651858.CD002014.pub3.

to understand why the focus seems to be on everything except the tightened muscles actually causing the pain.

Review of Scientific Research on Muscle Tension and Emotional Stress

There is not a lot of information available about the causation effect between emotional stress and muscular tension; however, there is a small body of scientific study that documents this important relationship to some degree. There are hundreds of medical studies worldwide that clearly identify emotional stress as the cause of muscular tension and pain, but most health-care providers who treat chronic pain don't consider that research in their treatment plans. In the section below there is a sampling of some of these studies. (Note: italics are mine for emphasis.)

In a study, authors focused on *physiological and muscle-tension* measures, differentiating work according to the level of mental demands. The results of this study concluded that mental demands on individuals were reflected by tension in in their arms, shoulder area, and forearm muscles.[12]

A study looking at fibromyalgia patients concluded that the patients showed elevated trapezius (triangular muscles extending over the back of the neck and shoulders) muscle activity in situations with imposed stress, including sympathetic (autonomic nervous system) activation and existing anticipatory stress.[13]

A study investigated physical, psychological, and social job characteristics as potential risk factors for complaints of pain in the arms,

---

12 . "The influence of mental load on muscle tension," *Ergonomics* 56, no. 7 (2013): 1125–1133, doi:10.1080/00140139.2013.798429.

13 . "Trapezius activity of fibromyalgia patients is enhanced in stressful situations, but is similar to healthy controls in a quiet naturalistic setting: a case-control study," *BMC Musculoskelet Disord* 14 (2013): 97, doi:10.1186/1471-2474-14-97.

neck, and shoulders (CANS). The findings implied that CANS therapy should be accompanied by improved job design from a psychological and social perspective and intervention aimed at decreasing short-term physical (muscular tension) and mental strain (need for recovery).[14]

A study looked at unfavorable psychosocial working conditions, which were believed to lead to stress and could be related to an increased risk of development of neck/shoulder symptoms. The study concluded that the results supported the idea that adverse psychosocial work conditions (high work demands) contribute to the development of neck/shoulder symptoms through the mechanism of stress-induced, sustained muscular activation.[15]

A study looked at anger management–style effects on CLBP patients. The study found that when patients were subjected to conditions of pain and mental stress, those patients who were allowed to express their feelings felt less of a pain effect than those patients who were required to suppress their feelings.[16]

A study found that increased *muscle tension in CBP patients may be responsible for the development and maintenance of chronic pain.* The study found that CBP patients showed patterns of higher muscular reactivity in the lower-back region.[17]

---

14 . "Office work and complaints of the arms, neck and shoulders: the role of job characteristics, muscular tension and need for recovery," *J Occup Health* 54, no. 4 (2012): 323–330, http://www.ncbi.nlm.nih.gov/pubmed/22673641.

15 . "Psychosocial work conditions, perceived stress, perceived muscular tension, and neck/shoulder symptoms among medical secretaries," *Int Arch Occup Environ Health*

16 . "Anger management style moderates effects of attention strategy during acute pain induction on physiological responses to subsequent mental stress and recovery: a comparison of chronic pain patients and healthy nonpatients," *Psychosom Med* 71, no. 4 (2009): 454–462, doi:10.1097/PSY.0b013e318199d97f.

17 "Muscular reactivity and specificity in chronic back pain patients." *Psychosom*

A study concluded that *patients with CLBP who suppress pain may detrimentally affect responses to the next event, particularly through prolonged muscle tension that may contribute to a cycle of pain-stress-pain.*[18]

A paper written by researchers concluded that anxiety makes depression worse, which is often accompanied by pain. Collectively, these factors can lead to a recurrent disorder and multiple medical symptoms with no discernible organic cause, and to chronic pain, even in response to an experience of minimal pain.[19]

This study looked at fibromyalgia syndrome (FMS) patients FMS patients and concluded that their pain perception occurred because they were not able to correct conditioned pain-producing muscle tension.[20]

In this case study, the researchers found that pain provoked by psychosocial stress factors may not be mediated through increased muscle activity (exercise).[21]

Med. Lombiewski JA, Tersek J, Rief W. 2008 Jan;70(1):125-31. Epub 2007 Dec 24.

18 . "The role of attentional strategies in moderating links between acute pain induction and subsequent psychological stress: evidence for symptom-specific reactivity among patients with chronic pain versus healthy nonpatients," *Emotion* 6, no. 2 (2006): 180–192, http://www.ncbi.nlm.nih.gov/pubmed/16768551.

19 . "From back pain to life-discontent: A holistic view of psychopathological contributions to pain," *Ann Med Interne* (Paris) 154, no. 4 (2003): 219–226, http://www.ncbi.nlm.nih.gov/pubmed/14593311.

20 . "The fibromyalgia syndrome as a manifestation of neuroticism?" *Z Rheumatol* 57, suppl. 2 (1998): 105–108, http://www.ncbi.nlm.nih.gov/pubmed/10025096.

21 . "Can stress-related shoulder and neck pain develop independently of muscle activity?" *Pain* 64, no. 2 (1996): 221–230, http://www.ncbi.nlm.nih.gov/pubmed/8740598.

This study concluded that results were consistent with the assumption that *psychological stress plays a role in musculoskeletal disorders.*[22]

In this study, the author concludes that a program of physician counseling and physical therapy is generally successful. *Pain syndromes involving the neck, shoulders, and low back are the result of a benign, reversible process in the musculature, which is psychosomatic in nature and has been called tension myositis.*[23]

Dr. John E. Sarno authored the last study listed above, and it was one of many of his clinical studies on the subject of tension and chronic pain.

When I realized that the causation between emotional stress and muscular tension had been studied and documented, I asked myself, *Why do we continue to treat a condition we know has its root cause in the mind with essentially* only *physical interventions?* It seems that part of the medical community understands that muscular tension and pain can be caused by emotions, but the part of the medical community that actually treats chronic back-neck-shoulder pain is unaware or does not take that into consideration. In the medical community there is clearly a line in the sand between doctors that treat the mind and doctors that treat the body. The problem for chronic-pain sufferers is that we need health-care providers who understand this complex relationship and can treat both sides of the patient, and those health-care practitioners are very difficult to find.

■ ■ ■

22 . "Psychophysiological stress and EMG activity of the trapezius muscle," *Int J Behav Med* 1, no. 4 (1994): 354–370, http://www.ncbi.nlm.nih.gov/pubmed/16250795.

23 . "Psychosomatic backache," *J Fam Pract* 5, no. 3 (1977): 353–357, http://www.ncbi.nlm.nih.gov/pubmed/143507.

Summary

EREIN I HAVE described my own crossing from sufferer of debilitating back and knee pain to someone who discovered a way to break a seemingly endless cycle of chronic pain. This adventure in healing has created a seismic shift in my understanding of mind-body synergy, health, fitness, and medicine. My life has been changed, and my vision of the future is now upbeat, positive, and full of joy. Throwing off the yoke of chronic pain has been an enlightening experience that I wish to bring to all who suffer as I did. I know that what has worked for me may not necessarily be the right solution for everyone, but it would be my great pleasure if these practices brought an end to chronic pain for many sufferers.

All creatures, human and nonhuman, are emotional by nature, and many of these emotions are handled outside of our conscious mind. Although we feel like we are managing the stresses of modern life effectively, we may be unaware of how our subconscious mind is emotionally overwhelmed. Our subconscious mind works in conjunction with the autonomic nervous system to find a way to dissipate negative emotional energy; it doesn't have any way to tell us "stop, things aren't going well; we need help." So that negative emotional energy is channeled to muscles in our body in the form of muscle contraction. The effect of those tightened muscles is a restriction in blood flow, which corresponds to a reduction in the oxygen flowing to that area of the body. When muscles and tissues are starved of oxygen, they respond with pain messages to the brain. Maybe that is the only way our subconscious mind can communicate to us that it is in crisis? I don't know, but if you have experienced chronic pain, you know it's a very strong message. As long as we continue to have negative emotions that are not well understood, mitigated, or dealt with, we are at risk for muscular pain that may become chronic.

Total Muscular Release can help to stop that cycle of negative emotions that leads to pain. Total Muscular Release has three phases: immersion, vigilance, and maintenance.

- Immersion (phase one): A practice of targeted muscle release.

- Vigilance (phase two): A practice of Complete Release TMR with directive self-talk.

- Maintenance (phase three): A phase that includes ongoing TMR on your entire body from time to time with directive self-talk, and extra targeted release work as necessary.

On the next page you will find a TMR Checklist. You can post this checklist somewhere handy to remind yourself about the items you'll need to follow through on each day to help you break your cycle of chronic pain.

☑	**TMR CHECKLIST**
	Believe: You can control your own muscular tension and, ultimately, your chronic pain.
	Practice Total Muscular Release: - Lie down comfortably, and begin to let your target muscles relax. - Completely drop your target muscles to the resting surface. - Relax the surrounding muscles connected to your target muscles. - Don't give up; repeat the release of your target muscles. - Continue to relax those muscles until you can it at will—do not quit. - Practice TMR as often as possible, wherever you are. - Practice TMR for your whole body from head to toe. - Practice Active TMR while moving, exercising, or doing any physical activity.
	Self-Talk: Tell your brain there will be NO MORE tension and NO MORE pain in your target muscles.
	Don't Hold Negative Emotions: Express your feelings. Negative emotions are OK, and can be dealt with properly.
	Review Your Emotional State Daily: Complete a review of your negative feelings and emotions each day. Observe it, own it, and when you can, let it go.

Our emotions are important in every sector of our lives, and they are keys to mind-body synergy. Emotions are like any other part of the body and deserve your attention. Be sure to review your emotions each day so that you can have understanding about your subconscious mind. Be honest with yourself about your emotions so you can clearly understand what is bothering you. Find ways to let go of negative or painful emotions that have no real meaning for you anymore. Throw away any old and useless emotional *junk* that no longer serves a purpose for you. Be kind to yourself, and give yourself some time during the day to meditate, pray, creatively visualize, or other contemplative, peaceful pursuits that are meaningful to you.

Stress—it is a killer. As described by the National Institute of Mental Health, there are at least three distinct types of stress, some of which may carry physical and mental health risks.

- Routine stress is stress related to the normal pressures of work, family, and other day-to-day responsibilities.
- Sudden stress is stress brought on by a sudden negative life change, such as the loss of a job, a divorce, illness, or other life event.
- Traumatic stress is stress related to an event like a major accident, war, assault, or a natural disaster that is experienced or where one is seriously hurt or in danger of being killed or dying.

Sometimes routine stress can cause changes in health, and that may be the hardest stress to recognize because the source is low-grade and constant, so the body gets no clear signal that it is time to turn it off and return to normal function. This continued strain on the body from routine stress can lead to serious health problems like depression, anxiety disorders, high blood pressure, heart disease, diabetes, and other illnesses. It is easy to say that we all have stress and there is not much we can do about it. It is true that stress is a constant in our lives, but it is imperative that you reduce your stress or at the very least understand it, own it, and deal with it. Failure to appropriately deal with stress will lead to a lifetime of chronic pain, disease, and illness. You can find a way to deal with your stress.

Exercise—Regarding exercise and breaking the cycle of chronic pain, I hesitate to talk about exercise in any manner that seems to be even the slightest bit negative, because we are living in a society in which the population becomes sicker and more obese with each passing year, but I will share a few things I have learned going through this process.

1. Exercise is important; it is good for you. You should vigorously exercise each day to keep yourself fit, capable of dealing with all that will come at you, and able to live a long, healthy, enjoyable life.
2. You do not need any special exercises, fitness classes, boot camps, workout routines, physical-fitness equipment or gear to overcome chronic pain that is caused by muscle tension.

When I was seeking a cure for my chronic pain, I tried a myriad of exercise regimes, and I did them faithfully morning and night, and more often at times. There were times when I was incapacitated with spasming muscles, and I would spend the day and night in bed exercising nearly every hour. Sometimes the training made me feel better, but in the back of my mind I was thinking, *Why do I have to spend so much time exercising day and night for so little reward?* It was an over-the-top way to have to live in order to keep my pain at bay for just a little while, but at the time it was all I had. I think you can imagine that finding a way to free myself from endless time-consuming and ineffective workouts felt like a gift, and it was.

During my long struggle, I read many books, and I watched hundreds of videos by skilled and well-meaning chiropractors, doctors, and physical therapists about how to relieve back pain. I now know that some of those activities will bring momentary periods of reduced pain. I would do the exercises; the muscles would be warmed with more circulation, and for some time there would be more oxygen supplied to muscles that were contracted, and the pain would subside. It was a short-term fix that I repeated as necessary, but it was not a cure, and the pain undoubtedly returned. In any case, I was thankful to everyone who took the time to provide information to help people like me, who were in so much pain. Sometimes that little bit of relief made life more bearable.

The cure will be in your ability to understand your emotions, deal with them, and master your TMR practice to break your cycle of tension. Reducing the amount of negative emotions in your subconscious can help lessen the pattern of tension-muscle contraction-lack of oxygen-pain in your back, neck, or shoulders. These negative feelings are very real to you, so acknowledge them, and own them so that they become less likely to loom as larger issues in your subconscious mind. Evaluate these emotional thoughts in your mind for a few minutes, and perhaps speak them out loud if that is helpful for you to articulate them better in your consciousness.

While you are performing these relaxation techniques, you may be thinking, *If I relax the muscles of my neck or back, won't I flop over or lose balance?* The answer is no. Your spinal column or neck is perfectly capable of holding itself up in a relaxed state. Does a dog or a cat or a horse worry about having good posture? No. They just let their bodies work naturally without any intervention. Many sectors of society ask us to change our posture: stand up straight, pull in the gut, hold the head up, pull back the shoulders, etc. It may be a family member, a teacher, or a well-meaning friend who suggests these stiff and unnatural postures, which are not always good for us in the long run. A reasonable posture is certainly good for the body, but as we get older, all of these artificial poses can cause us tension and pain. If we have awareness of these types of messages that we are receiving from the world, we can hopefully avoid additional tension and pain in the future.

Chronic pain is a loop that serves a purpose for our subconscious mind, but it do us harm over time. Thankfully, any negative path in the body can be changed or turned into a more positive one. If you are suffering from chronic pain caused by muscular tension and have read this book, I hope you understand that you now have all the training you need, as well as the innate ability within yourself to free yourself from the trap of tension-based chronic pain. Once you break that *tension-muscle contraction-lack of oxygen-pain cycle*, you will be able to master your chronic pain.

Practicing Total Muscular Release can help you stop the pain loop by circumventing the tension in the first place. Once you are able to relax muscles that have been the source of your chronic pain, and you are free from chronic pain, you will be safe in the knowledge that you can manage any new tension-inducing situation that comes up in the future. Taking control of your tension will reduce and hopefully eliminate your pain and allow you to be at peace again.

Mind-body synergy is not simply an important concept in health and healing but also the most critical component for resolving emotional tension-based pain. There are as many different types of pain as there are people in the world. Each individual is unique, and his or her path to health and healing is special and singular. The course of TMR treatment that I took for myself and have outlined in this book is certainly my own, and I cannot say that it will work for everyone. However, my understanding of my tension and chronic pain is that it is not unique or different from the tension and pain experienced by many others. Medical science has brought us many amazing advancements and has been a great boon to humanity in many ways, but clearly it does not have all the answers for everyone.

The Dalai Lama has said, "If we do nothing to restrain our angry, spiteful, and malicious thoughts and emotions, happiness will elude us," which of course is wise advice for all of us and applies well to the subject of tension-based chronic pain. Human beings are blessed with so many outstanding qualities and attributes which allow us to do spectacular things in the world. I have the greatest hope that the words written here will help some people break their cycles of tension and pain, and allow them to experience joyful lives.

■ ■ ■

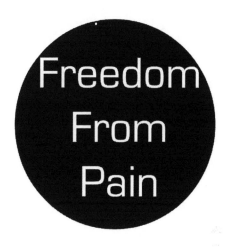

Afterword

M
Y *BACK STORY* is told. It's a simple tale with a truly amazing payoff for me—an absolutely, positively amazing transformative experience that occurred in a very short period of time. I did not need any magic, pain pills, therapy, doctors, or other intervention except my own mind and body. To this day, I feel fully relaxed in even the most tension-inducing situations. I take on life without fear of chronic pain.

Have I entered a trance, a beguiled Zen-like state, or gained some superpowers that have allowed me to divert tension like some sort of Wonder Woman? No. I feel the same negative emotions that all people feel each day as I cope with work, family, friends, and all the other aspects of being human. I have discovered a way to stop those negative emotions from becoming physical tension. Having knowledge of TMR, while continuing to recognize and acknowledge my negative emotions, has freed me. Once the muscles were released from the tension, and the oxygen levels returned to normal, my pain was gone.

For someone with chronic pain, letting go of the tension in those muscles that have been causing the pain for a long time must seem like an impossible task. Until I created this method, I was unable to do anything about it, but I'm sure anyone can learn these skills and break the cycle of tension-based chronic pain. Hopefully you will see the strength of this powerful form of mind-body control and soon be able to control your emotions, tension, and pain.

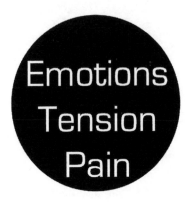

Like many of you who suffer from chronic neck-back-shoulder pain, I had tried numerous different doctors, chiropractors, therapies, pain relievers, exercises, etc., but I found no long-term relief from any of those modalities. One day I stumbled upon the idea of Total Muscular Release, and after a short period of time I developed a method that resolved my chronic pain. It was a simple concept that helped me greatly, and after I saw its effects I knew that it could help others as well. This ability is in all of us, and that makes us all special healers, indeed. We need to seek it, understand it, work with it, and believe in ourselves. I wish each of you health, happiness, and a pain-free life.

■ ■ ■

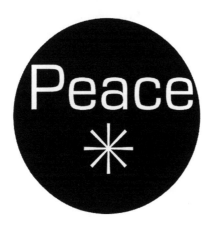

Further Reading

READ ONE OR more of Dr. John Sarno's books in order to understand his concepts of tension myositis syndrome (TMS):

Healing Back Pain: The Mind-Body Connection (2001)

The Mindbody Prescription: Healing the Body, Healing the Pain (1999)

The Divided Mind (2009)

Mind Over Back Pain (1986)

Look for the first Whitehall Study of British civil servants in 1967-compared mortality of people in the highly stratified environment of the British Civil Service. There was a follow-up study as well. It showed that, among British civil servants, mortality was higher among those in the lower grade than the higher grade. The more senior one was in the employment hierarchy, the longer one might expect to live as compared to people in lower employment grades.

A helpful publication by the National Institute of Mental Health is *Adult Stress—Frequently Asked Questions: How It Affects Your Health and What You Can Do About It* (http://www.nimh.nih.gov/health/publications/stress/stress_factsheet_ln.pdf).

Stress: Portrait of a Killer (2008 documentary)

"Stress is not a state of mind...it's measurable and dangerous, and humans can't seem to find their off switch."

These words of warning come from renowned author and award-winning neurobiologist Robert Sapolsky in the documentary *Stress: Portrait of a Killer*. The film, jointly produced by National Geographic and Stanford University (where Dr. Sapolsky is a professor and scholar), shows just how dangerous prolonged stress can be.

In addition, you may want to read about relaxation techniques for the body and relaxing breathing exercises as well.

If you feel that you have serious emotional problems that may be causing your tension, you should seek advice from a mental-health professional.

About the Author

SHERRI OBERMARK IS an artist and writer living and working in Cincinnati, Ohio. She enjoys life with her husband, son, family, friends, and three red tabby cats.

Made in the USA
San Bernardino, CA
01 February 2019